Critical Care in
DERMATOLOGY

Critical Care in DERMATOLOGY

Editors

Arun C Inamadar MD DVD
Professor and Head
Department of Dermatology, Venereology and Leprosy
Sri BM Patil Medical College, Hospital and Research Center
BLDE University
Bijapur, Karnataka, India

Aparna Palit MD (PGIMER, Chandigarh)
Professor
Department of Dermatology, Venereology and Leprosy
Sri BM Patil Medical College, Hospital and Research Center
BLDE University
Bijapur, Karnataka, India

Foreword
Jean Paul Ortonne

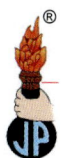

JAYPEE BROTHERS MEDICAL PUBLISHERS (P) LTD
New Delhi • London • Philadelphia • Panama

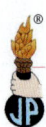

Jaypee Brothers Medical Publishers (P) Ltd

Headquarters

Jaypee Brothers Medical Publishers (P) Ltd
4838/24, Ansari Road, Daryaganj
New Delhi 110 002, India
Phone: +91-11-43574357
Fax: +91-11-43574314
Email: jaypee@jaypeebrothers.com

Overseas Offices

J.P. Medical Ltd
83 Victoria Street, London
SW1H 0HW (UK)
Phone: +44-2031708910
Fax: +02-03-0086180
Email: info@jpmedpub.com

Jaypee-Highlights Medical Publishers Inc.
City of Knowledge, Bld. 237, Clayton
Panama City, Panama
Phone: + 507-301-0496
Fax: + 507-301-0499
Email: cservice@jphmedical.com

Jaypee Brothers Medical Publishers Ltd
The Bourse
111 South Independence Mall East
Suite 835, Philadelphia, PA 19106, USA
Phone: + 267-519-9789
Email: joe.rusko@jaypeebrothers.com

Jaypee Brothers Medical Publishers (P) Ltd
17/1-B Babar Road, Block-B, Shaymali
Mohammadpur, Dhaka-1207
Bangladesh
Mobile: +08801912003485
Email: jaypeedhaka@gmail.com

Jaypee Brothers Medical Publishers (P) Ltd
Shorakhute, Kathmandu
Nepal
Phone: +00977-9841528578
Email: jaypee.nepal@gmail.com

Website: www.jaypeebrothers.com
Website: www.jaypeedigital.com

© 2013, Jaypee Brothers Medical Publishers

All rights reserved. No part of this book may be reproduced in any form or by any means without the prior permission of the publisher.

Inquiries for bulk sales may be solicited at: jaypee@jaypeebrothers.com

This book has been published in good faith that the contents provided by the contributors contained herein are original, and is intended for educational purposes only. While every effort is made to ensure accuracy of information, the publisher and the editors specifically disclaim any damage, liability, or loss incurred, directly or indirectly, from the use or application of any of the contents of this work. If not specifically stated, all figures and tables are courtesy of the editors. Where appropriate, the readers should consult with a specialist or contact the manufacturer of the drug or device.

Critical Care in Dermatology

First Edition: **2013**

ISBN : 978-93-5090-285-1

Printed at: Ajanta Offset & Packagings Ltd., New Delhi

Dedicated to
The pioneer dermatologists who
propagated the concept of
'Acute Skin Failure'
and
'Intensive Care in Dermatology'

Shuster
Irvine
Rene Touraine
Terrance Ryan

Contributors

Abhay Mani Martin
Consultant Dermatologist
Baby Memorial Hospital
Indira Gandhi Road
Kozhikode-673004, Kerala, India
E-mail: abhaydoc@gmail.com

Aparna Palit
Professor
Department of Dermatology,
Venereology and Leprosy
Sri B.M. Patil Medical College
Hospital and Research Center
BLDE University
Bijapur-586103, Karnataka, India
E-mail: apalit2011@gmail.com

Arun C Inamadar
Professor and Head
Department of Dermatology,
Venereology and Leprosy
Sri B.M. Patil Medical College
Hospital and Research Center
BLDE University
Bijapur-586103, Karnataka, India
E-mail: aruninamadar@gmail.com

BV Peerapur
Professor and Head
Department of Microbiology
Raichur Institute of Medical Sciences
Raichur, Karnataka, India
E-mail: Peerapur_2003@yahoo.co.in

Kumar GV
Assistant Professor
Department of Pediatrics
Sri Siddhartha Medical College
Tumkur, Karnataka-572107, India
E-mail: kumargowripura@yahoo.co.in

Laxmi Nair
Former Professor and Head
Department of Dermatology
Calicut Medical College
Kerala, India
'Krishnakripa', Kavu Nagar
Chevayur PO, Calicut-673017
Kerala, India
E-mail: laxminairv@gmail.com

Murlidhar Rajagopalan
Senior Consultant and
Coordinator, Dermatology
Apollo Hospitals
Chennai, Tamil Nadu, India
No-25, Ground Floor
Beach Residency
1st Seaward Road, Valmiki Nagar
Chennai-600041 Tamil Nadu, India
E-mail: murlilata@gmail.com

Nazeer Ahmed K
Professor
Department of Anesthesiology
and Critical Care
Al-Ameen Medical College and
Hospital
Bijapur-586108, Karnataka, India
E-mail: nazeer8@yahoo.co.in

Ragunatha S
Associatie Professor
Department of Dermatology,
Venereology and Leprosy
Sri Siddhartha Medical College
Tumkur, Karnataka-572107, India
E-mail: drragus@yahoo.co.in

Vineet Kaur
Consultant Dermatologist
The Skin Institute, Varanasi
Member, Board of Directors
International Skincare Nursing
Group, B-34, Brij Enclave
Varanasi-221005
Uttar Pradesh, India
E-mail: drvineet11@gmail.com

Foreword

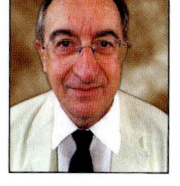

The book 'Critical Care in Dermatology' includes all the aspects of intensive care in Dermatology; in the 11 chapters of this book general principles of management of dermatological emergencies are explained in lucid manner.

The tables, figures, photos and the flow charts are very well presented. This new book will be an addition to dermatology literature. Dermatologists will not only have the opportunity to know the classic diagnostic procedures and management of skin disorders but also to recognise, evaluate and treat emergencies in the specialty.

Two Indian dermatologists, Arun C Inamadar MD DVD, and Aparna Palit MD, will propagate this intensive care in dermatology and most dermatologists will be proficient in providing critical care.

Prof Jean Paul Ortonne
Chair, Department of Dermatology
Professor, Hospital L'Archet
Nice University, France
Editor, Journal of European Academy of
Dermatology & Venereology (JEADV)

Preface

The subject 'Dermatology' has the image of an outpatient specialty with trivial fatality, among the medical fraternity. The term "dermatologic emergency" is often regarded as an oxymoron in the medical world. Dermatology does involve emergencies, despite the general impression that patients with dermatological illnesses never die and never get well, and the specialty is all about applying various colored lotions!

Emergency medicine or critical care medicine is a well-established subspecialty of internal medicine. Of late the concept of 'critical care in dermatology' is gaining importance as the concept of 'acute skin failure' has been increasingly recognized and the need for 'Dermatology Intensive Care Unit' is felt.

There can be serious, life-threatening skin conditions or complication of diseases or therapy that require immediate intervention in critical care setup. It is necessary to acquire skills in 'emergency dermatology', where a dermatologist's right decision and intervention can make an important difference between life and death. According to Dr Wolf, 'The topic of dermatologic emergencies is indeed broad and covers almost all the fields of modern medicine'. Special situations like pregnancy, neonate and associated metabolic disorders demand critical care.

Most dermatologists are not proficient in providing critical care. There is scarcity of reference book or literature devoted to this topic. This book is an attempt to fill the gap and present all the necessary inputs for better management of critically ill patients due to dermatological illnesses. We hope that this book will contribute to a better image of dermatology as a dynamic and innovative subject.

We thank all the authors for their contribution to this book. We are thankful to Jaypee Brothers Medical Publishers for their neat work.

Arun C Inamadar
Aparna Palit

Acknowledgments

We are thankful to the Department of Anesthesia and Department of Medicine, Sri BM Patil Medical College, Hospital and Research Center, BLDE University, Bijapur, Karnataka, India, for their contribution to this book.

Contents

Chapter 1: Dermatological Emergencies: General Considerations   1

Arun C Inamadar

- *Introduction and Definition   1*
- *Dermatological Emergencies: Magnitude of the Problem   2*
- *Classification   4*
- *Approach to a Patient with Dermatological Emergency   4*
- *History   6*
- *Acute Skin Failure: An Overview   8*
- *General Principles of Management of Dermatological Emergencies   11*

Chapter 2: Dermatological Emergencies   13

Aparna Palit

- *Erythroderma   15*
- *Psoriasis   19*
- *Severe Cutaneous Adverse Drug Reactions   22*
- *Anaphylaxis   35*
- *Vascular Disorders   38*
- *Collagen Vascular Disorders   55*
- *Complicated Vascular Tumors   57*
- *Vesiculobullous Disorders   60*
- *Infections   67*
- *Bacterial Toxin Mediated Illnesses   82*
- *Reactions in Leprosy   89*
- *Bites/Stings/Venom   93*
- *Metabolic Disorders   100*
- *Drug-Induced Cutaneous Necrosis   104*
- *Acute Graft Versus Host Disease   109*

Chapter 3: Fluid, Electrolyte and Nutrition Therapy in Dermatological Emergencies   114

Ragunatha S, Kumar GV

- *Body Fluid Compartments   115*
- *Fluid, Electrolyte Disturbances and Protein Loss in Acute Skin Failure   115*
- *Fluid, Electrolyte and Nutritional Therapy in Dermatological Emergencies   116*

- *Fluid Resuscitation in Patients with Ten 117*
- *Fluid and Electrolyte Therapy in Erythroderma 120*
- *Nutritional Supplementation in Patients with Dermatological Emergencies 121*

Chapter 4: Procedures and Techniques in Dermatological Emergencies   125
Nazeer Ahmed K
- *Vital Signs and Monitoring 125*
- *Universal Precautions 126*
- *Procedures and Maneuvers 127*
- *Vascular Access 128*
- *Airway Access/Maintenance 136*
- *Nasogastric Access 143*
- *Transurethral Catheterization 146*
- *Cardiopulmonary Resuscitation 149*
- *Acknowledgement 154*

Chapter 5: Diagnostic Procedures in Critical Care Set Up   156
BV Peerapur
- *Blood Culture 157*
- *Pus Sample Collection 158*
- *Specimen Collection from Skin 158*
- *Specimen Collection from Throat and Mouth 159*
- *Specimen Collection from Rectum 160*
- *Bedside Estimation of Bleeding Time and Clotting Time 160*

Chapter 6: Nursing Care in Dermatological Emergencies   163
Vineet Kaur
- *Skin Care Nursing in Non-Dermatological Critically Ill Patients 164*
- *Nursing Care of ohe Skin in Dermatological Emergencies 169*

Chapter 7: Dermatology Intensive Care Unit (DICU)   177
Arun C Inamadar
- *Concept of Intensive Care and Intensive Care Unit 177*
- *Admission Criteria for DICU 178*
- *Multidisciplinary Approach in Patients Admitted in DICU 179*
- *How to Set Up DICU? 179*
- *Instruments and Equipments 180*
- *Emergency Drugs 183*
- *Skills to be Acquired by Dermatologists 184*

Chapter 8: Drugs Used in Dermatological Emergencies   186
Arun C Inamadar, Abhay Mani Martin
- *Classification   186*
- *Adrenaline   187*
- *Dopamine   189*
- *Dobutamine   189*
- *Frusemide   189*
- *Atropine   190*
- *Colloids and Crystalloids   190*
- *Sodium Bicarbonate   192*
- *Calcium Gluconate   193*
- *Oxygen Therapy   194*
- *Corticosteroids   194*
- *Cyclosporine   198*
- *Methotrexate   199*
- *Cyclophosphamide   202*
- *Vincristine   204*

Chapter 9: Rescue Therapy in Dermatology   206
Arun C Inamadar, Murlidhar Rajagopalan
- *Cyclosporine as Rescue Therapy   207*
- *Infliximab as Rescue Therapy   208*
- *Corticosteroid as Rescue Therapy   209*
- *Rescue Therapy in Methotrexate Toxicity   209*
- *Rescue Therapy in Dapsone Induced Methemoglobinemia   211*
- *Rescue Therapy in Cyclophosphamide Induced Bladder Toxicity   212*
- *Other Indications of Rescue Therapy in Dermatology   212*

Chapter 10: Dermatological Drug Therapy in Challenging Clinical Scenarios   214
Ragunatha S
- *Dermatological Drug Therapy in Patients with Renal Impairment   215*
- *Dermatological Drug Therapy in Patients with Hepatic Impairment   219*

Chapter 11: Drugs in Pregnancy and Lactation   229
Laxmi Nair
- *Physiological Changes in Pregnancy and their Effect on Pharmacokinetics   230*
- *Drug Dosing in Pregnancy   232*
- *Prenatal Development and Relationship with Maternal Drug Intake   232*

- *Pharmacokinetics of Drugs Ingested by the Mother in the Fetus* 233
- *Drug Categorization During Pregnancy* 234
- *Drug Prescription in Lactating Women* 236
- *Monitoring and Management Principles* 237

Appendix 243

Index 253

chapter 1

Dermatological Emergencies: General Considerations

Arun C Inamadar

- Dermatological emergencies: magnitude of the problem
- Classification
- Approach to a patient with dermatological emergency
- History
- Acute skin failure: an overview
- General principles of management of dermatological emergencies

INTRODUCTION AND DEFINITION

Emergency medicine or critical care medicine is a well-established subspecialty of internal medicine. Of late the concept of 'emergency dermatology/critical care in dermatology' is gaining importance in day-to-day dermatology practice. With introduction and innovation of newer molecules for the management of various dermatological conditions, gone are the days of using GV lotion alone! Special situations like pregnancy, neonate and associated metabolic disorders and comorbid conditions demand critical care.

The explosion of new medical knowledge and resultant technologies for patient care has changed the scope of dermatology. Dermatologists play a key role in diagnosis and management of skin disorders in intensive care units and emergency departments as well as in the more traditional outpatient arena. All practicing dermatologists must now not only be familiar with the classic dermatological disorders but also be able to recognize, evaluate, and treat emergencies in dermatology.

We must salute the forethought of Shuster, the great dermatologist, who dealt with 'systemic manifestations of cutaneous disorders' way back in 1967. His treatise on this subject is the basis of coinage of the term 'acute skin failure' and rationale for intensive care in dermatology.

The concept of dermatologic intensive care unit (DICU) is also gaining wider acceptance, as it has become mandatory to manage patients with acute skin failure, e.g. toxic epidermal necrolysis (TEN), etc., in an aseptic environment with multispecialty consultation and all the necessary gadgets for maintaining vitals, fluid and electrolyte balance. It is almost akin to 'burn ward'. In fact dermatological emergencies are still managed in burn ward in many parts of the world.

Burn injury affects skin integrity and partial thickness burns usually blister. In patients with burn, the barrier function against fluid loss is totally damaged. Burn injury is a dynamic process that peaks at about 3 days after the thermal trauma. TEN is a widespread immunological injury leading to epidermal loss in sheets leaving a dark red oozing dermis as compared to the burn injury which involves the deep dermis too. TEN carries worse prognosis than burns of the same extent because of systemic involvement like hepatitis, hematological abnormalities, and subclinical interstitial edema culminating into frank pulmonary edema. Required quantity of fluid replacement also differs in both the conditions. Hence, it was right by Professor Rene Touraine to shove a unit devoted to the intensive care of dermatological diseases way back in 1976 amidst the criticism he faced from his colleagues.

The word 'emergency' may be defined as follows:
- An unforeseen combination of circumstances or the resulting state that calls for immediate action. *(Webster's medical desk dictionary)*
- A sudden serious and dangerous event or situation which needs immediate action to deal with it. *(Oxford dictionary)*

In the medical field 'emergency' stands for 'immediate action' to tackle the unforeseen (expected or unexpected) complication of the disease process or those arising from use of the therapeutic agents.

DERMATOLOGICAL EMERGENCIES: MAGNITUDE OF THE PROBLEM

It is often a challenge for a dermatologist to provide effective care for more serious, life-threatening conditions that require immediate intervention. Skin conditions that may require intensive care are relatively rare. Hence, it is difficult for individual dermatologists to gain experience of managing such cases. The magnitude of the problem can be gauged from the list of certain dermatological conditions in which mortality ranges from minimal to very high (**Table 1.1**).

In a secondary analysis of the Intensive Care National Audit & Research Centre (ICNARC) Case Mix Programme Database (Critical care 2008), data was extracted for 476,224 admissions to 178 intensive care units (ICU) in England, Wales and Northern Ireland participating in the programme over the time period from December 1995 to September 2006. They identified admissions with dermatological conditions from the primary and secondary reasons for admission to ICU, and total 2,245 dermatological admissions were identified. Conditions included infections (e.g. cellulitis, necrotizing fasciitis), dermatological malignancies, and acute skin failure (e.g. Stevens–

Table 1.1: Mortality associated with various dermatological emergencies

Dermatologic emergency	Mortality (%)
Neonatal erythroderma	16%
SSSS	< 0.5%

TSS
  Menstrual
  Nonmenstrual
	
	13–15%
	03–05%

Meningococcemia with DIC	>50%
Necrotizing fasciitis	59%
Rocky mountain spotted fever (RMSF)	30–70%
Neonatal varicella	20–23%
Neonatal HSV	04–85%
Dengue shock syndrome	40–50%
Candidiasis in neonates	08–40%
Kasabach-Merritt phenomenon	20–30%
Purpura fulminans	50–100%
Kawasaki disease	0.1–02%
Sclerema neonatorum	50–100%

Drug reactions
  SJS
  DHS
  TEN
	
	05%
	10–38%
	30%

Anaphylaxis	<10%
Hereditary angioedema	02%
Catastrophic antiphospholipid antibody syndrome	50%
Acute GVHD (moderate to severe)	50%

Johnson syndrome [SJS], TEN, and autoimmune blistering diseases). These represented 0.47% of all ICU admissions, or approximately 2.1 dermatological admissions/ICU/year. Overall mortality was 28.1% in the ICU and 40% in hospital. Length of stay in intensive care was longest for those with acute skin failure (median 4.7 days for ICU survivors and 5.1 days for ICU non-survivors). They identified patients who not only required intensive care, but also dermatological care. Such patients (UK ICU population) had high mortality rate and long ICU stay, similar to other acute medical conditions. This highlights the importance of skin failure as a distinct entity comparable to other organ system failure.

The incidence of SJS and TEN are better characterized, and have been estimated at 0.4 to 1.2 and 1.2 to 6 million person years, respectively. There is a slightly increased risk in females. Mortality from erythema multiforme (EM) does not exist but may occur in 10% for patients with SJS, approximately 30% for patients with SJS/TEN-overlap and almost 50% for patients with TEN. For SJS, SJS/TEN-overlap and TEN together the mortality rate is almost 25%. In order to evaluate the mortality due to SJS/TEN, time of death in relation to the onset of the reaction, age of the patient, underlying diseases and the amount of skin detachment have to be considered. Medications most commonly associated with these conditions are sulfonamide and non-sulfonamide antibiotics, anticonvulsants and nonsteroidal anti-inflammatory drugs. Of these medications, sulfonamides have the highest risk. In the era of HIV/AIDS and increased incidence of associated oppurtunistic infections, the list of drugs causing severe cutaneous drug reaction is expanding. Abacavir hypersensitivity is a well-known entity. Nevirapine (antiretroviral) and lamotrigine (antiepileptic) are the newer drugs added to the list of drugs causing SJS/TEN.

In an overview of the major causes responsible for erythroderma from 13 reviews quoted in Mark Lebwohl's 'Difficult diagnoses in dermatology', approximately half of all the cases were secondary to primary dermatological condition (eczema, psoriasis, pemphigus foliaceus, lichen planus and pityriasis rubra pilaris), with remaining cases occurring due to systemic drug reactions, malignancy and of undetermined etiology. In a study involving 91 patients with erythroderma, the disease specific mortality was 18%.

Ten to 25% of angioedema patients are due to angiotensin-converting-enzyme inhibitor (ACEI) therapy, occurring in 1–2/1000 new users.

■ CLASSIFICATION

Emergencies in dermatology may result from:
1. Primary skin diseases
2. Systemic disorders with cutaneous manifestations.

Prompt recognition and diagnosis with subsequent appropriate treatment might improve the prognosis in both the categories. **Table 1.2** presents the list of conditions which may result in dermatological emergency.

■ APPROACH TO A PATIENT WITH DERMATOLOGICAL EMERGENCY

Given the extensive list of causes of 'acute skin failure' and 'erythroderma' requiring the critical care, it is imperative that the clinicians have an organized approach to the diagnosis of these conditions. It should cover the history, physical examination and laboratory evaluation.

Table 1.2: Conditions resulting in dermatological emergency

1. **Erythroderma**
2. **Psoriasis:**
    i. Psoriatic erythroderma
    ii. Acute generalized pustular psoriasis of Von Zumbusch
3. **Severe cutaneous adverse drug reactions:**
    i. SJS-TEN
    ii. Drug hypersensitivity syndrome
    iii. Urticaria/Angioedema
    iv. Serum sickness
    v. Drug-induced anaphylaxis
4. **Anaphylaxis**
5. **Vascular disorders:**
    i. Urticaria/angioedema
    ii. Purpura fulminans
    iii. Antiphospholipid antibody syndrome
    iv. Calciphylaxis
    v. Kawasaki disease
6. **Collagen vascular disorder:**
    i. Acute cutaneous lupus erythematosus
7. **Complicated vascular tumors:**
    i. Kasabach-Merritt phenomenon
    ii. Multifocal/diffuse neonatal hemangiomatosis
8. **Vesiculobullous disorders:**
    i. Genetic blistering disorders
    ii. Immunobullous disorders
9. **Infections:**
    i. Necrotizing fasciitis
    ii. Meningococcemia
    iii. Disseminated gonococcal infection
    iv. Rocky mountain spotted fever
    v. Dengue hemorrhagic fever and dengue shock syndrome
10. **Bacterial toxin mediated illnesses:**
    i. Staphylococcal scalded skin syndrome
    ii. Toxic shock syndrome
    iii. Scombroid fish poisoning
11. **Leprosy reactions:**
    i. Acute neuritis with nerve abscess/impending palsy
    ii. Severe form of type 2 reaction
12. **Bites/stings/venom:**
    i. Bite by insects of *Hymenoptera* species (bees, wasps, fire ants)
    ii. Spider envenomation (black widow spider, brown recluse spider)
    iii. Tick paralysis
    iv. Jellyfish, sea anemones and coral stings

Contd...

Contd...

13. Metabolic disorders:
i. Neonatal biotin deficiency
ii. Acrodermatitis enteropathica
14. Drug induced cutaneous necrosis:
i. Warfarin/coumarin necrosis
ii. Heparin necrosis
iii. Tissue necrosis due to vasopressors
15. Acute graft vs. host disease

History

- Prenatal history
- Onset and course
- Associated abnormalities
- Provocation by sunlight
- Topical exposure to potential allergen
- Systemically administered drug before the onset of the condition.

Physical Examination

- Extent of erythroderma/body surface area (BSA) of involvement
- Areas of accentuation
- Associated cutaneous changes (scalding, pustules and crusting)
- Nail/hair/other congenital abnormalities
- Color of the skin
  - Pallor: atopic dermatitis (AD)
  - Salmon red hue: pityriasis rubra pilaris (PRP)
  - Orange hue: chronic lymphocytic leukemia
  - Bluish hue: lichenoid reaction.
- Pattern of scaling
  - Ichthyosiform scaling: congenital ichthyosiform erythroderma (CIE), atopic dermatitis (AD), sarcoidosis, lymphoma, leukemia
- Vesicles/bullae
  - Acute eczema
  - Pemphigus foliaceus.
  - Drug eruptions
  - Epidermolytic hyperkeratosis
  - Graft vs. host disease (GVHD)
- Ulceration of the skin
  - Lymphoma
  - Leukemia
  - Histoplasmosis
- Nail plate pitting (> 20 pittings on fingernails is suggestive of psoriasis)
- Oral manifestations (lichen planus, drug eruption, histoplasmosis, Reiter's disease)

- Ocular manifestations (AD, Reiter's disease, sarcoidosis, histoplasmosis)
- Joint manifestations (psoriasis, drug reactions, Reiter's disease, sarcoidosis)
- Massive/asymptomatic lymphadenopathy
  - Lymphoma, leukemia, drug rash, sarcoidosis
- Splenomegaly
  - Lymphoma/leukemia, drug reaction, sarcoidosis, histoplasmosis, Reiter's disease and GVHD

Laboratory Evaluation

- Stain and culture for bacterial/fungal infections
- Calcium levels (hypercalcemia: sarcoidosis)
- Peripheral smear for Sezary cells (15 or > Sezary cells/100 lymphocytes: Sezary syndrome and actinic reticuloid)
- Leukemic cells in peripheral smear
- Screening for metabolic disorders
- Blood urea nitrogen (BUN)/serum creatinine
- Random blood sugar (RBS)/lipid profile
- Serum electrolytes assay.

Skin Biopsy

Serial/multiple skin biopsies from representative areas: histopathological (HPE) and immunofluorescence (IMF) study.

Prognostic Criteria

SCORTEN **(Table 1.3)** is calculated as evaluation tool for prediction of prognosis of toxic epidemal necrolysis (TEN). Simplified acute physiological score (SAPS) is well correlated to the mortality rate of patients with acute skin failure. Indicators of poor prognosis are:

- Age of the patient (extremes of the age)
- Extent of skin lesions
- Neutropenia
- Elevated blood urea
- Administration of high dose of steroids

Chest X-ray

Chest X-ray may be abnormal in sarcoidosis, histoplasmosis or malignancies. In drug induced erythroderma, patient may be screened with chest X-ray to rule out active pulmonary tuberculosis, and it may help in planning the treatment. Pulmonary involvement is the most severe systemic complication of TEN. An early chest X-ray would detect subclinical interstitial edema.

Table 1.3: Severity illness score for TEN

Risk factors	
Age	>40 years
Concurrent illness	Malignancy
Epidermal detachment	>30% body surface area
Serum urea	>28 mg /dl (>10 mmol / L)
Blood glucose level	> 252 mg / dl (> 14 mmol / L)
Sodium bicarbonate level	< 20 mEq / L (< 20 mmol / L)
Heart rate	> 120 beats / minute

Number of risk factors: 0-1, mortality rate 3.2%; 2, mortality rate 12.1%; 3, mortality rate 35.3%; 4, mortality rate 58.3%; ≥ 5, mortality rate 90%.

ACUTE SKIN FAILURE: AN OVERVIEW

Shuster was the first dermatologist to study the systemic effects of extensive skin diseases. Functions of skin are manifold ranging from forming a simple mechanical barrier to complex role as an immunological outpost and storehouse of hormonal activity. Alteration in these functions of skin due to extensive skin ailments may lead to significant morbidity and certain amount of mortality by different ways akin to acute failure of vital organs like kidney and liver. Prototype disease for understanding of acute skin failure (ASF) is TEN.

Evolution of the concept of ASF is based on the following:
- Loss or derangement in the expected functions of skin.
- Physiological and/or pathological consequences of dermatological conditions ranging from hereditary disorders of cornifications ending in erythroderma to drug induced TEN.

Irvine (1991) was the first person to define the skin failure as '*loss of normal temperature control with inability to maintain the core body temperature and failure to prevent percutaneous loss of fluid, electrolytes and protein with resulting imbalance, and failure of mechanical barrier to prevent penetration of foreign materials*' and proposed that it was a real entity comparable to any other major organ system dysfunction.

The principal pathomechanism of ASF has been summarized in **Figure 1.1**.

ASF is comparable to any other major organ system dysfunction because of the following consequences:
- Fluid and electrolyte imbalance
- Protein and calorie loss
- Impaired thermoregulation
- Alteration in immunological function and infection
- Systemic involvement.

Fluid, Electrolyte and Protein Loss/Imbalance

Exudation of fluid, proteins and electrolytes occur due to loss of the outermost cover of the body. An average loss of 3 to 4 liters of fluid is estimated to occur in TEN involving 50% of the BSA. Significant protein loss is not seen with intact skin but occurs only when it is inflamed. Increased albumin excretion, increased catabolism and reduced synthesis may lead to hypoalbuminemia. All these losses may end up in hypotension and consequent renal failure.

Thermoregulation

Impaired control of skin blood flow and inability to sweat is observed in patients with extensive skin disease leading to impaired thermoregulation. Hypothermia may set in with shivering and calorie loss. A sudden drop in the patient's temperature may be the first sign of the ensuing sepsis.

Infection

Infection may be the major cause of mortality in extensive skin loss or involvement. Susceptibility to infection is due to impaired immune response, loss of barrier function of the skin, administration of steroids and use of other immunosuppressive drugs as therapeutic modality for primary skin conditions. Intravenous line through the affected skin may add to the problem. Fever itself may not be an indicator of secondary infection or sepsis.

Following may be the signs of sepsis:
- Sudden drop in blood pressure
- Drop in temperature
- An altered consciousness
- Oliguria.

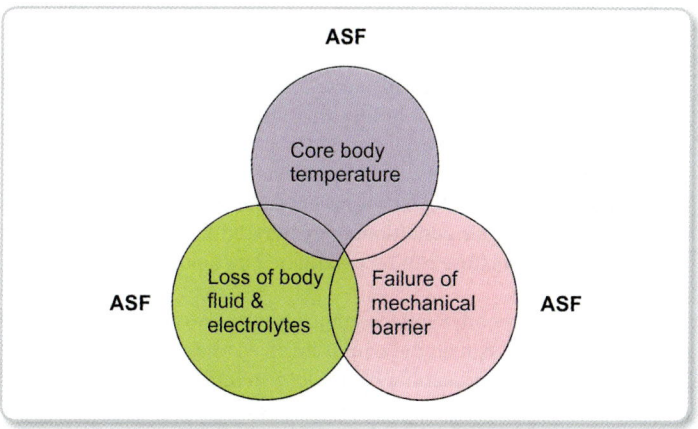

Figure 1.1: Principal pathomechanism involved in acute skin failure

Cardiovascular Complications

There may be left ventricular failure (LVF) because of increased blood flow through the skin and consequent increased cardiac output. Pre-existing ischemic heart disease in an elderly patient may lead to precipitation of pulmonary edema and may initiate respiratory distress syndrome (RDS). Interleukin-1 and Tumor necrosis factor-α mediated capillary leak in severe generalized pustular psoriasis has been reported to result RDS. Prolonged immobilization may be a predisposing factor for venous thrombosis.

Management of Acute Skin Failure

Management in DICU setup is desirable due to the anticipated complications and related mortality as follows:
- Secondary infection and septicemia
- Fluid and electrolyte imbalance
- Hypovolemic shosck
- Cardiovascular failure
- Pulmonary edema
- Disseminated intravascular coagulation.

Regular skin swab from different body sites should be taken to know the organism, which may be the cause of infection and to decide upon appropriate antibiotic. Antibiotics are indicated if there is sign of sepsis. Some authors administer broad spectrum antibiotics empirically, if there is leukopenia associated with TEN.

In the event of inadequate oral intake, nasogastric feeding is advised (in patients without any evidence of malabsorption). If intravenous fluid has to be administered, peripheral line should be through the uninvolved skin. Intravenous fluids administered at similar rate like patients with burn in a patient with ASF may end up with pulmonary edema. Hence, it is important to estimate fluid loss and requirement in each individual patient with ASF by repeated clinical assessment. In the first 24 hours, the fluid administration may be estimated according to the extent of skin loss.

Temperature control is an important issue in ASF. The room temperature should be increased to prevent shivering and calorie loss. This may be achieved by air conditioners or infrared light in resource poor setup. Optimum moisture can be maintained by boiling a large kettle in the corner of room.

Noninvasive hemodynamic monitoring by pulse oximeter is preferred especially when the skin on the arms is involved (difficult to record blood pressure with sphygmomanometer). Close monitoring of urine output and vital parameters is essential.

GENERAL PRINCIPLES OF MANAGEMENT OF DERMATOLOGICAL EMERGENCIES

Management of ASF depends upon the causative disease. These must be treated in DICU setup to improve the outcome. Therapies to address the 'loss of barrier function', 'fluid loss', 'impaired thermoregulation' and 'effective control of infection' are mandatory to reduce the morbidity and mortality. Hourly monitoring of vitals, precise watch on patient's hemodynamics and culture/sensitivity data is essential. Nutritional supplementation in the form of high calorie protein rich alimentation by tube feeding, judicial use of antibiotics at the earliest direct or indirect signs of sepsis (avoiding prophylactic use of antibiotics) and managing the energy loss by maintaining the optimum thermal environment are the additional requirements in the effective management of ASF.

Multidisciplinary approach is called for to address all the known causes of mortality like secondary infection and septicemia, fluid and electrolyte imbalance, hypovolemic shock, cardiovascular failure, pulmonary edema and disseminated intravascular coagulation. Physicians, surgeons, pediatricians and anesthetists play important role in the management of patients with ASF. These goals can be achieved in a setup of DICU. Dermatologists need to know when and where to utilize the cross-consultation of fellow medical colleagues. It is also mandatory to know the basic minimum about the procedures necessary for revival of the patient in case need arises.

Role of Physician and Pediatrician

- Consultation for systemic involvement
- Consultation for pre-existing systemic disease
- Consultation for advise regarding alternative drugs for pre-existing systemic disease (especially in cases with drug reactions)
- Consultation for fluid and electrolyte therapy
- Consultation for nutritional therapy
- Consultation for medical complications and emergencies.

Role of Surgeon

- Consultation for surgical complications and emergencies
- Venesection
- Wound debridement.

Role of Anesthetist

- Endotracheal intubation
- Central venous catheterization
- Arterial catheterization
- Mechanical ventilation.

In conclusion, patients with dermatological emergencies deserve special attention and management protocol. Establishment of DICU is a positive step towards achieving this goal. Organization of a dedicated and coordinated multi-specialty member team is the essential initial step for establishment of DICU. Various stages of establishment of DICU has been discussed in chapter 7.

■ SUGGESTED FURTHER READING

1. Dunnill MGS, Handfield-Jones SE, Treacher D, Mcgibbon DH. Dermatology in the intensive care unit. Br J Dermatol 1995;132:226–35.
2. Freiman A, Borsuk D, Sasseville D. Dermatologic emergencies. CMAJ 2005;173:1318–19.
3. George SM, Harrison DA, Welch CA, Nolan KM, Friedmann PS. Dermatological conditions in intensive care: a secondary analysis of the Intensive Care National Audit & Research Centre (ICNARC) Case Mix Programme Database. Critical Care 2008;12:S1.
4. Gerull R, Nelle M, Schaible T. Toxic epidermal necrolysis and Stevens-Johnson syndrome: A review. Crit Care Med 2011;39:1521–32.
5. Inamadar AC, Palit A. Acute skin failure: concept, causes, consequences and care. Indian J Dermatol Venereol Leprol 2005;71:379–85.
6. Irvine C. 'Skin failure'—a real entity: discussion paper. J R Soc Med 1991;84:412–3.
7. Lehnhardt M, Jafari HJ, Druecke D, Steinstraesser L, Steinau HU, Klatte W, et al. A qualitative and quantitative analysis of protein loss in human burn wounds. Burns 2005;31:159–67.
8. Roujeau JC, Revuz J. Intensive care in dermatology. In: Champion RH, Pye RJ, editors. Recent advances in dermatology, No 8. Edinburgh: Churchill Livingstone; 1990. p-85–100.
9. Shuster S. Systemic eFfects of skin disease. Lancet 1967;1:907–12.
10. Sigurdsson V, Toonstra J, Hezemans-Boer M, van Vloten WA. Erythroderma. A clinical and follow-up study of 102 patients, with special emphasis on survival. J Am Acad Dermatol 1996;35:53–7.
11. Vonderheid E. Chronic generalized erythroderma. In: Lebwohl M, editor. Difficult diagnoses in dermatology. New York: Churchill Livingstone; 1988.p-89–100.

chapter 2

Dermatological Emergencies

Aparna Palit

- Erythroderma
- Psoriasis
- Severe cutaneous adverse drug reactions
- Anaphylaxis
- Vascular disorders
- Collagen vascular disorders
- Complicated vascular tumors
- Vesiculobullous disorders
- Infections
- Bacterial toxin mediated illnesses
- Reactions in leprosy
- Bites/stings/venom
- Metabolic disorders
- Drug-induced cutaneous necrosis
- Acute graft versus host disease

INTRODUCTION

Though traditionally believed as a lighter medical branch, unwarranted situations may arise occasionally in dermatology practice at par with major medical branches like cardiology or neurology. Table 1.2 in first chapter presents the list of the conditions which may result in emergency situation for dermatologists. In the following section these conditions will be discussed briefly in the background of emergency situation. Some of these conditions give rise to acute skin failure which should be managed in an intensive care unit (ICU), designed to fulfill the requirement of these patients with special provisions for temperature and humidity control (dermatological intensive care unit, DICU). However, such an arrangement is an unreality in majority of the health care setup. Alternatively, these patients may be managed in an advanced burn care unit. In some other conditions resulting in dermatological emergencies, there is major systemic involvement and in the course of illness, these patients may require intense cardiovascular and pulmonary monitoring and resuscitation. These patients may be managed in a general ICU with a multi-specialty approach.

Table 2.1: Important causes of erythroderma with differential diagnosis

Causes of erythroderma	Clinical diagnostic clue	Other differentiating features
Ichthyosis & related syndromes	Present since or soon after birth. Adherent scales.	History of collodion membrane at birth may be present Family history may be positive.
Psoriasis	Typical psoriasiform plaque in early stage; scales are loose, coarse and silvery	Typical nail changes like pitting and oil drop sign— Arthritis.
Pityriasis rubra pilaris (PRP)	Islands of normal skin within salmon colored erythema. Follicular papules on dorsal surface of fingers, elbows, wrists, PRP sandal on palms & soles	Histopathology showing alternate orthokeratosis and parakeratosis oriented in both horizontal and vertical directions.
Inflammatory disorder • **Atopic dermatitis (AD)**	Fulfilling diagnostic criteria for AD	History of recurrent episodes with typical distribution. Personal or family history of other atopic disorders.
• **Seborrhoeic dermatitis**	Yellowish greasy scale involving seborrhoeic areas predominantly	History of recurrent episodes of seborrhoeic dermatitis.
• **Airborne contact dermatitis**	Acute/subacute/chronic dermatitis with or without photo exacerbation.	Prior history of contact dermatitis due to plant allergens/cement, etc.
Pemphigus foliaceous	Superficial erosions with collarettes of scale. Nikolsky's sign may be positive	Positive Tzanck smear, subcorneal split in histopathology.
Infections • **SSSS**	Positive Nikolsky's sign, skin tenderness	
• **Scarlet fever** • **Generalized congenital candidiasis**		

Contd...

Contd...

Causes of erythroderma	Clinical diagnostic clue	Other differentiating features
Infestations • Norweigian scabies	Intense pruritus in the background of immunosuppressed state	Demonstration of mite under microscope
Drug induced • DHS	Systemic involvement like hepatitis, pneumonitis, nephritis	History of drug intake Altered liver function tests
Malignancy associated • Sézary syndrome	Leonine facies in long-standing cases	Presence of Sézary cells in peripheral blood (>20%)
Dermatomyositis	Heliotrope rash, poikiloderma, Gottron's papules, proximal muscle weakness	Raised muscle enzymes
Sarcoidosis	Ichthyosiform erythroderma	Histopathology showing sarcoidal granuloma

ERYTHRODERMA

Introduction

Erythroderma denotes generalized erythema, scaling and induration involving approximately > 90% of the body surface area. It is a morphological description which may be the end result of various dermatological conditions. Various important causes of erythroderma have been presented in **Table 2.1**.

Why the Disease is an Emergency?

An erythrodermic patient is susceptible to acute skin failure and following related complications:
- Temperature dysregulation
- Dehydration
- Electrolyte imbalance
- Protein depletion
- Infection and septicemia
- High output cardiac failure
- Adult respiratory distress syndrome (ARDS).

Population at Risk

Barring hereditary disorders and atopic dermatitis, erythroderma mostly affects middle aged individuals (>45 years). Males are more common sufferers of erythroderma due to any cause.

Clinical Presentation

In a patient suffering from a primary illness, rapidly spreading generalized erythema, followed by scaling is the initial presentation. In an established patient of erythroderma, there is erythema, scaling and induration involving >90% of body surface area (**Figures 2.1A to F**). Due to a taut skin there may be ectropion, eclabium, everted nostrils and flexion contracture of limb joints. Skin may show deep fissures at places. In erythroderma of some duration there may be exaggerated skin folds and shedding of scalp hair, eyelashes and nails. Generalized lymphadenopathy may be present and patient may develop diarrhea resulting from associated enteropathy.

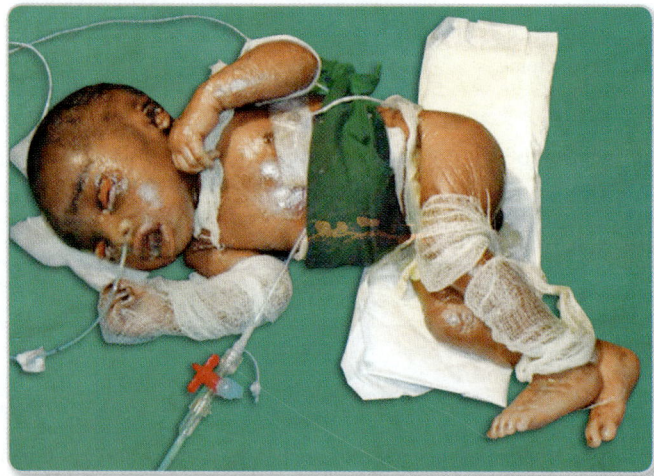

Figure 2.1A: Collodion baby

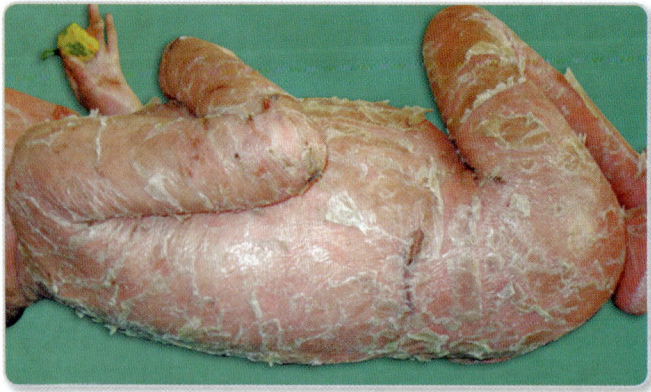

Figure 2.1B: Non-bullous ichthyosiform erythroderma (NBIE)

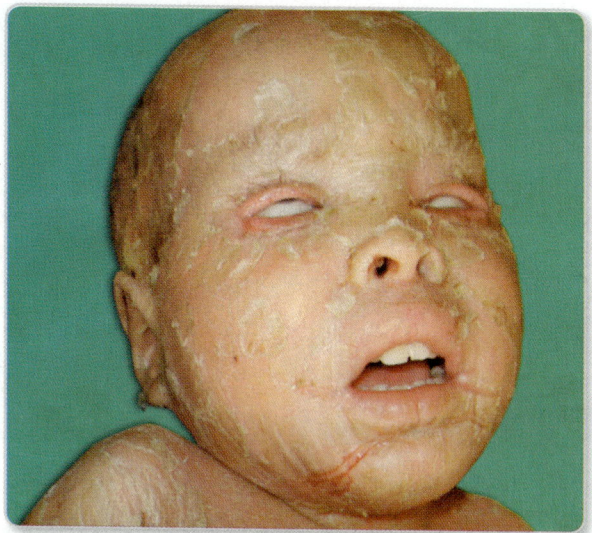

Figure 2.1C: Ectropion, eclabium and everted nostrils in a case of NBIE. Note deep fissure on the chin

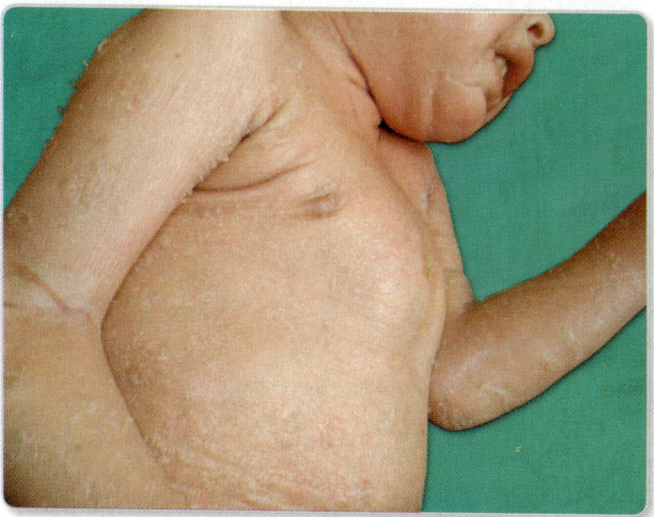

Figure 2.1D: NBIE following treatment with systemic isotretinoin

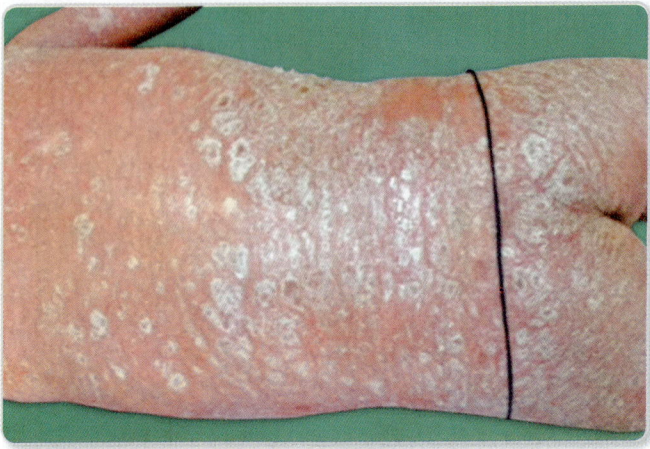

Figure 2.1E: Psoriatic erythroderma

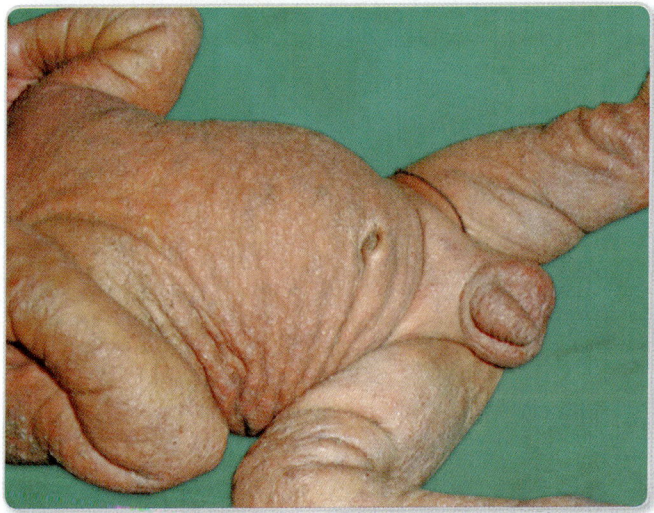

Figure 2.1F: Infantile erythroderma due to Norwegian scabies. Note exaggerated skin folds

Clinical Clues

Clinical diagnostic clues to various causes of erythroderma have been presented in **Table 2.1**.

Rapid Laboratory Diagnostic Methods

Skin biopsy and histopathological examination is done to establish the underlying cause of erythroderma.

When hospitalized, routine monitoring of the patients needs various laboratory investigations, as follows:
- Serum electrolytes
- Blood urea, serum creatinine
- Complete hemogram
- Serum albumin
- Repeated culture and sensitivity test from skin discharge.

Differential Diagnosis (Table 2.1)

Management

Patients with mild erythroderma of short duration may be managed at home in an isolated room in a warm and humidified environment. However, with slightest hint of cardiopulmonary compromise or evidence of infection, the patient must be shifted to hospital. Patients with erythroderma should be managed in a DICU.

Management of erythroderma requires a comprehensive approach:
- Maintenance of optimum environmental temperature and humidity
- Barrier nursing
- Strict intake/output chart
- Supplementation of fluid, electrolytes and vitamins as and when indicated
- High protein diet
- Antibiotics if there is evidence of infection
- Sedative oral antihistamine in presence of pruritus
- Topical application of bland emollients
- Specific treatment of underlying cause (e.g. psoriasis/atopic dermatitis/ichthyosis, etc.).

PSORIASIS

A. Psoriatic erythroderma
B. Acute generalized pustular psoriasis of von Zumbusch

Psoriatic Erythroderma

Discussed in erythroderma section.

Acute Generalized Pustular Psoriasis of von Zumbusch

Introduction

It is a generalized variant of pustular psoriasis, which occurs in a known patient of chronic plaque/any other morphological variant of psoriasis. The patient may develop pustulation due to any provocating factor, most commonly after sudden withdrawal of topical or systemic corticosteroid. It is an uncommon variant of psoriasis.

Why the Disease is an Emergency?

Acute generalized pustular psoriasis is associated with very high rate of complications and may lead to sudden death. Following complications may arise during the course of the disease:
- Severe hypoalbuminemia
- Hypocalcemia and tetany
- Oligemia and acute renal tubular necrosis
- Deep vein thrombosis and pulmonary embolism
- Malabsorption
- Acute generalized pustular psoriasis of pregnancy is associated with severe constitutional symptoms like fever, vomiting, diarrhea, delirium, and the patient may die due to tetany, cardiac failure or renal failure.

Population at Risk
- Patients on treatment with certain drugs (**Table 2.2**)
- Psoriasis patients during pregnancy
- Psoriasis patients with hypoparathyroidism and hypocalcemia
- Individuals with certain HLA types; HLA-B27, HLA-CW1.

Clinical Presentation

The generalized pustular eruption is preceded by intense burning sensation, erythema and skin tenderness and thereafter high fever and malaise. The patient may develop numerous pinpoint pustules at the margin of existing skin lesions (pustular collarettes) or it may be generalized (**Figures 2.2A and B**). There may be repeated crops of lesions with bouts of fever and cutaneous erythema and in an established case there is confluence of pustules to form lakes of pus. There is remission of individual bouts with dried up pustules and exfoliation. During an acute episode of severe pustulation, patient may develop erythroderma.

Table 2.2: Drugs precipitating pustular psoriasis

1. Topical therapy
• Potent corticosteroid (addition/sudden withdrawal)
• Coal tar
• Anthralin
2. Systemic therapy
• Corticosteroids (sudden withdrawal)
• Ciclosporin (sudden withdrawal)
• Salicylates
• Phenylbutazone & Oxyphenbutazone
• Iodide (cough formula)
• Progesterone
• Terbinafine
• Bupropion (for cessation of smoking)

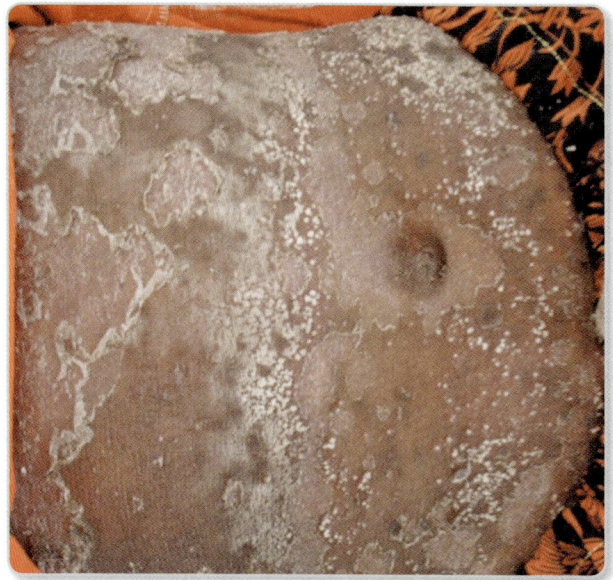

Figure 2.2A: Acute generalized pustular psoriasis (von Zumbusch)

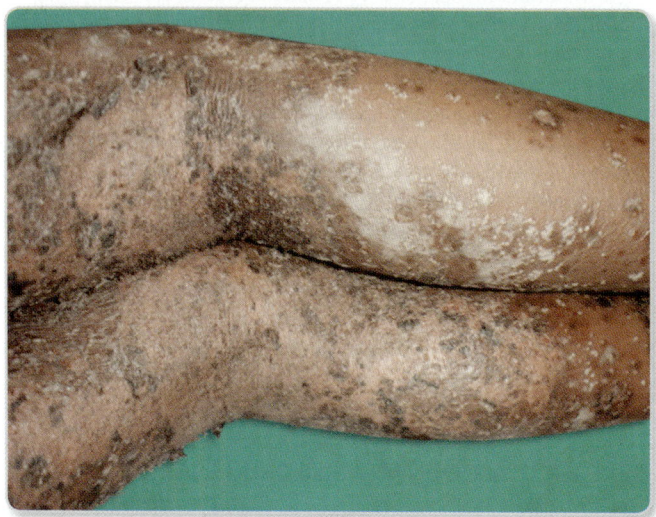

Figure 2.2B: Pustular psoriasis with "lakes of pus"

Clinical Clues

- In known patients with psoriasis, crops of pustular lesions should alert the clinician to consider the possibility of pustular psoriasis.

- Preceding warning symptoms like burning sensation, erythema, fever, skin tenderness.
- Presence of 'lakes of pus' in an established case.
- Geographic tongue or fissured tongue may be associated.

Rapid Laboratory Diagnostic Methods

In case of diagnostic difficulty, skin biopsy and histopathological examination confirms the diagnosis. Gram stained smear from pustules reveal polymorphonuclear cells without organism. Following laboratory tests may be done:
- Complete hemogram, which may reveal initial absolute lymphopenia followed by polymorphonuclear leukocytosis.
- Raised ESR.
- Serum protein reveals low plasma albumin.
- Low serum calcium.

Differential Diagnosis
- Acute generalized exanthematous pustulosis.

Management

Patient should be admitted in a DICU for management. Detailed history taking is important to rule out any precipitating factor, especially drugs and any such drug must be withdrawn. Symptomatic conservative treatment with mild sedative, fluid replacement and high protein diet may help to overcome the acute episode. Only bland emollients should be used for skin care. Systemic therapy is comprised of the following:
- Acitretin (1 mg/kg/day), to overcome the acute stage and thereafter 0.5 to 0.75 mg/kg/day, to maintain the control.
- PUVA therapy, small doses initially, gradually increasing dose.
- Combination therapy with acitretin and PUVA.
- Methotrexate (0.3 mg/kg, total 7.5–10 mg weekly) administered IM/IV, to avoid the risk of malabsorption if administered through oral route.
- Ciclosporin at a high dose (9–12 mg/kg/day).
- Parenteral corticosteroid, when there is severe metabolic complications which require urgent control.
- In pregnant patients, systemic corticosteroids/ciclosporin.

SEVERE CUTANEOUS ADVERSE DRUG REACTIONS

Severe adverse drug reactions (ADR) are associated with high mortality constituting 4th–6th leading cause of inpatient death. No age is immune to develop drug reaction but it is relatively rare at extremes of ages, i.e. pediatric and geriatric age group. Generally women are more susceptible to develop ADR as compared to men. The risk of cutaneous ADR (CADR) increases steadily with age (adults > adolescents > children); among the elderly it is probably related to higher number of concurrently prescribed drugs rather than the influence of age. Immunosuppressed patients including those with HIV infection are more prone to develop CADR. History and temporal relationship with drug intake is helpful in the diagnosis of CADRs. Provocation test (challenge test) with the suspected culprit drug proves the diagnosis but absolutely contraindicated in severe drug reactions. Immediate withdrawal of the inflicting drug is mandatory for all types of drug reactions.

Severe cutaneous adverse drug reactions include:
A. Stevens Johnson syndrome (SJS)/SJS-Toxic epidermal necrolysis overlap (SJS-TEN)/Toxic epidermal necrolysis (TEN)
B. Drug hypersensitivity syndrome (DHS)
C. Drug-induced urticaria and/or angioedema
D. Serum sickness
E. Drug-induced anaphylaxis (to be discussed in anaphylaxis section).

SJS/SJS-TEN/TEN

Introduction

SJS, SJS-TEN and TEN are disorders characterized by widespread epidermal and mucosal necrosis, mostly induced by drug administration or sometimes precipitated by exposure to chemicals or infection. During the prodromal phase, there is fever, cough, myalgia, conjunctival congestion, sore mouth and a maculopapular rash simulating viral illness. Soon thereafter the epidermal necrosis supervenes, initially in the form of target lesions and may progress rapidly to result in sheets of epidermal separation. Overall mortality associated with SJS is around 5%, which is escalated up to 30% in TEN.

A patient with fully developed TEN simulates burn injury and requires similar degree of care either in DICU or in a burn unit. The basic difference between the two conditions is that burn is an acute insult which remains non-progressive thereafter; whereas, SJS-TEN group of disorders continue to progress till the provoking factor is identified and withdrawn (drug) or adequately treated (infection). In drug-induced cases, even after withdrawal of the drug, the disease may progress for few more days because of presence of its metabolites in body. Hence, patients with SJS-TEN group of disorders require more diligent observation and careful monitoring.

Why the Disease is an Emergency?

The mortality rate associated with SJS-TEN is as high as 25 to 30%. In SJS and TEN, there is widespread loss of cutaneous barrier, giving rise to acute skin failure. Secondary infection may lead to septicemia, a leading cause of death in these patients. Other causes of death in these patients are gastrointestinal bleeding, aspiration pneumonia and pulmonary embolism.

Population at Risk

Young adults are the common sufferers of SJS-TEN spectrum of illness and men are twice more commonly affected than women. Children are prone for infection (*Mycoplasma pneumoniae*) induced SJS in addition to drugs. In patients with comorbid factors like underlying diabetes, hypertension, malignancies and immunosuppressive therapy, severity of the disease and related complications are augmented. Patients with HIV infection and AIDS are at thousand times higher risk of developing TEN as compared to normal population.

Clinical Presentation

Target skin lesions (typical/atypical) and mucosal erythema or erosions (> 1 site) are the presenting features of this group of disorders (**Figures 2.3A and B**). Extent of body surface area (BSA) involvement determines the spectrum of the disease, (<10% = SJS, 10–30% = SJS-TEN overlap, >30% = TEN). Widespread denudation of skin without preceding target lesions may be the presenting feature in case of TEN (**Figures 2.4A and B**). Nikolsky's sign is positive (**Figure 2.4C**).

Clinical Clues

Patients may complain of a generalized burning sensation and/or skin pain prior to the development of target lesions. Hemorrhagic crust of the

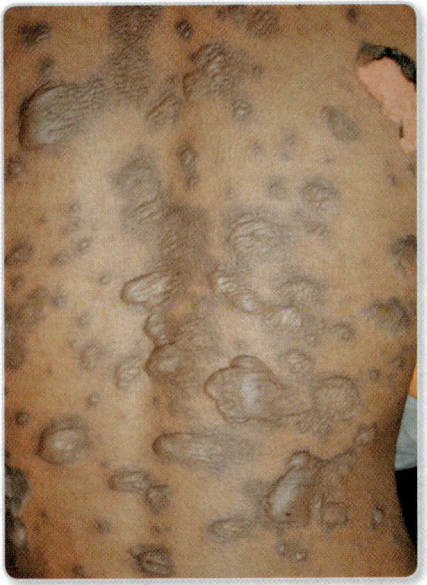

Figure 2.3A: Stevens Johnson syndrome

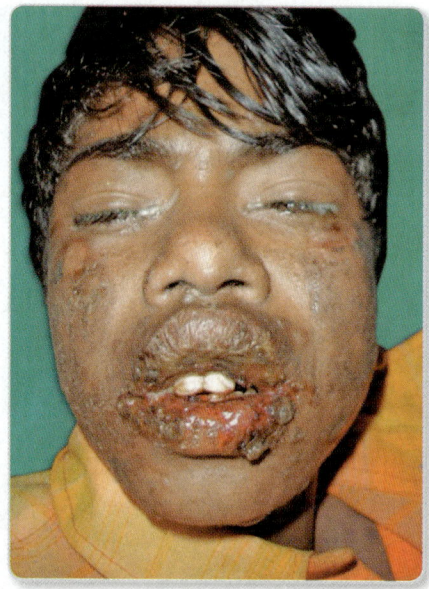

Figure 2.3B: Hemorrhagic crusts on lips in a patient with Stevens-Johnson syndrome

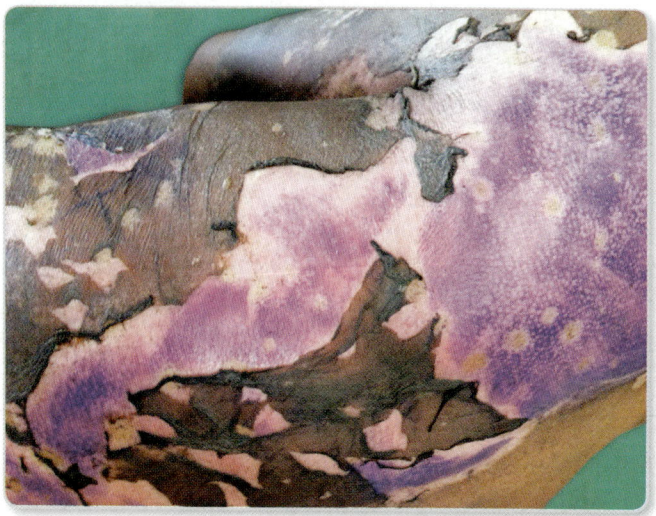

Figure 2.4A: Toxic epidermal necrolysis with widespread epidermal detachment

lips is a pointer to the diagnosis of SJS/TEN spectrum of disorder even in the absence of target lesions. Diffuse erythema and skin tenderness are the early features of TEN, before the onset of epidermal detachment.

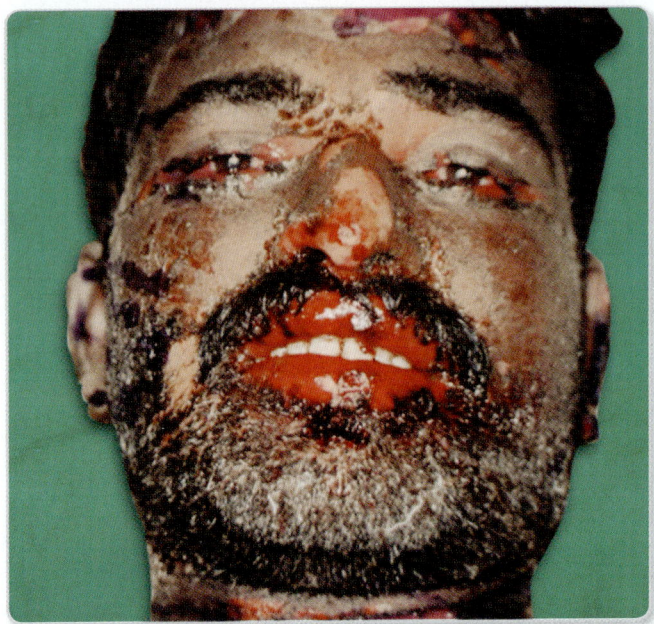

Figure 2.4B: Mucosal involvement in toxic epidermal necrolysis

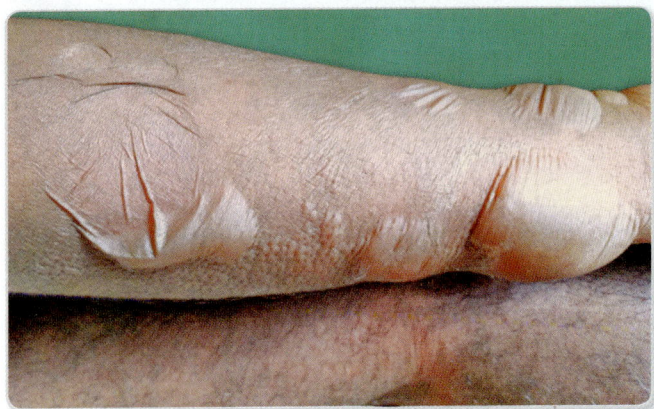

Figure 2.4C: Positive Nikolsky's sign in a patient with TEN

Rapid Laboratory Diagnostic Methods

In case of diagnostic confusion in patients with SJS and TEN, Tzanck smear may be done from freshly denuded area, which demonstrates few necrotic keratinocyte and plenty of inflammatory cells. Frozen section histopathological examination of the skin may be helpful in rapid and early diagnosis.

Other laboratory investigations for monitoring of the patient include:

- Total and differential leukocyte count (lymphopenia, neutropenia in 30% cases)
- Platelet count (thrombocytopenia in 15% cases)
- Blood sugar (often increased)
- Blood urea/serum creatinine (often increased)
- Serum aminotransferases (slight increase in 50% cases)
- Urine microscopy
- Microbial analysis from following materials:
  - pus/discharge from skin
  - blood (if septicemia is suspected)
  - mucosal swab
  - urine
  - intravenous canula tip and urinary catheter tip
- Chest X-ray (interstitial edema in early stage, pneumonia in 30% cases)
- In presence of acute skin failure, serum electrolytes are to be monitored regularly.

Differential Diagnosis

- Erythema multiforme minor (in the initial stage)
- Staphylococcal scalded skin syndrome
- Immunobullous disorders.

Management

These patients must be admitted in DICU for close monitoring. On 1st day of admission, SCORTEN prognostic score must be calculated for all patients to assess the individual prognosis and thereafter repeated periodically.

General Measures
- Immediate withdrawal of the drug.
- Aseptic environment (box isolation) and barrier nursing.
- Maintenance of optimum room temperature (around 30°C) to prevent hypothermia. This may be achieved by using heat shields/infrared lamps.
- Air-fluidized bed.
- Bladder catheterization (in male patients condom catheterization is preferable).
- Intravenous line/central venous catheterization (to be done preferably through uninvolved areas of skin). The indwelling lines must be scrutinized everyday for evidence of infection and should be replaced every 3rd day.
- Intake/output chart.

- Supplementation of fluid, (approx. 5–7 liters in first 24 hours, a combination of macromolecules and saline) electrolytes and vitamins as and when indicated.
- Gentle nasogastric tube insertion if the patient is unable to take orally and high calorie, high protein, liquid diet is administered at regular intervals. If patient is able to swallow, oral intake is encouraged with liquid/semisolid diet, comprised of high protein.
- Skin care: daily bath/sponging; local cleaning of erosions followed by topical application of 1% gentian violet lotion over raw areas and dressing with paraffin soaked gauze pieces. Intact bullae should be drained by multiple small incisions and the skin is allowed to rest on the floor of the lesion (natural dressing). Biological dressings may be used for eroded areas, if available.
- Mucosal care: Regular examination of mucous membrane (oral, ocular, genital in females) to prevent complications.

  Maintenance of oral hygiene.

  Removal of oral and nasal debris.

  Regular instillation of artificial tear and antibiotic drops (in presence of infection) in the eyes. Eyelids are covered with eye pads if closure is incomplete. Early ocular adhesions are gently disrupted using a glass rod.

  Dressing and lubrication of vaginal erosions (prevents synechiae formation).
- Prompt intubation and ventilatory support at the earliest sign of ARDS.

Therapy
- Antibiotics, if there is evidence of infection; following may be the indicators of occult infection:
  - rigor
  - fever or sudden hypothermia
  - hypotension
  - decreased urinary output
  - deterioration of respiration and level of consciousness
  - deterioration of diabetic control.
- Parenteral H_2-blocker to prevent stress ulcers.
- Analgesia (IV bolus dose of opioid analogue tramadol) as and when indicated.
- Anxiolytic/sedative drug may be used if the patient is apprehensive.
- Though controversial, short course (3–5 days) of parenteral systemic steroid may be used, if the patient's disease is in the evolution phase (eruption of many new lesions) or there is intense inflammation/edema of skin lesions and/or mucosa (lips, buccal mucosa).
- Specific treatment includes high dose intravenous immunoglobulin (IVIg), adult dosage being 1 to 2 mg/kg/day for 3 to 4 days. It has to be started early in the course of the disease to achieve the beneficial effect.

- All patients with SJS/TEN must be provided with a warning card (with mention to avoid the causative drug and other related drugs) which they must carry while seeking medical consultation.

Drug Hypersensitivity Syndrome

Introduction

Drug hypersensitivity syndrome (DHS) is a clinical triad of fever, skin rash and visceral involvement due to exposure to a drug. There are various other names to designate this disorder including the acronyms DRESS and DIDMOHS. Common drugs causing DHS are anticonvulsants, sulfonamides, INH, phenylbutazone, allopurinol, nevirapine and abacavir. DHS occurs during the first course of the drug but not with the first dose and an interval of 1 to 8 weeks is characteristic. Prolonged disease course and slow resolution is usual in DHS. Recurrences are common and such episodes are more severe.

Why the Disease is an Emergency?

Patients with drug hypersensitivity syndrome usually present with erythroderma and related complications. There is associated hepatitis which may progress to fulminant hepatic failure, rapidly developing hepatic encephalopathy. There may be multisystemic involvement, like nephritis, pneumonitis, myocarditis and encephalitis. The mortality associated with DHS ranges around 10–38%.

Population at Risk

Women are more at risk of developing DHS. Patients with slow-acetylator status develop this disorder more frequently. With co-morbid conditions (e.g. alcoholic liver disease, infective hepatitis, pulmonary tuberculosis, chronic glomerulonephritis), the severity of the illness is perpetuated.

Clinical Presentation

Generalized maculopapular rash which may progress to exfoliative dermatitis and facial edema are the initial features of drug hypersensitivity syndrome (**Figure 2.5**). It is associated with icterus, generalized lymphadenopathy and hepatomegaly. Rarely skin lesions may be vesicular or vesiculo-bullous, simulating SJS. Cutaneous features may be subtle (transient skin rash) with predominant visceral involvement.

Clinical Clues

Icterus, hepatomegaly and generalized lymphadenopathy in a patient with generalized skin rash or exfoliative dermatitis are the clinical pointers to the diagnosis of DHS.

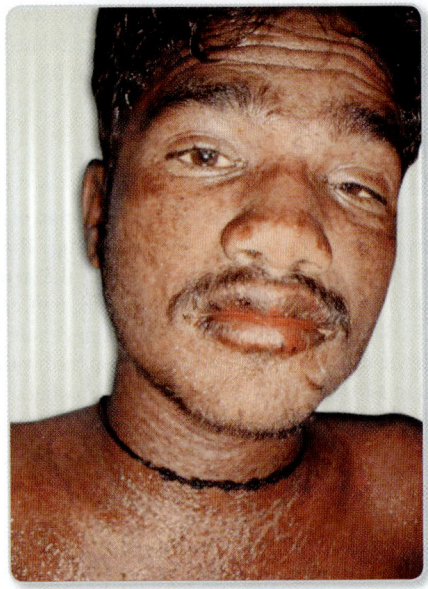

Figure 2.5: Drug hypersensitivity syndrome due to phenytoin

Rapid Laboratory Diagnostic Methods
- Differential leukocyte count and absolute eosinophil count (to demonstrate eosinophilia, present in 90% cases).
- Peripheral blood smear (atypical lymphocytes and mononucleosis is detected in 40% cases).
- Liver function test (raised bilirubin and hepatic enzymes).
- Viral serology (HBsAg and HCV) to rule out infective hepatitis.
- Chest X-ray to rule out pulmonary involvement.
- Estimation of eosinophil cationic protein, which is raised in acute stage of the disease and helps in monitoring.

Differential Diagnosis
- Viral hepatitis
- Obstructive jaundice
- Maculopapular drug rash
- Viral exanthem.

Management
Immediate withdrawal of the drug.
Mild cutaneous lesions are to be managed symptomatically.
- In presence of erythroderma, patient should be managed in DICU with:
    - Aseptic environment and barrier nursing
    - Strict intake/output chart

- Supplementation of fluid, electrolytes and vitamins as and when indicated
- High protein diet
- Antibiotics if there is evidence of infection
• High dose systemic corticosteroid (0.5–1 mg/kg) is the mainstay of therapy in presence of severe visceral involvement, which results in symptomatic improvement as well as gradual normalization of the laboratory parameters (e.g. elevated hepatic enzymes). The dose should be tapered gradually to minimize the chances of recurrence.
• Other modalities used to treat DHS are interferon-γ (chronic course), IVIg and ciclosporin.
• All patients with DHS must be provided with a warning card (with mention to avoid the causative drug and other related drugs) which they must carry while seeking medical consultation.

Drug-Induced Urticaria and/or Angioedema

Introduction

Drug-induced urticaria is seen in 0.16% of hospital inpatients and it is the second commonest CADR following maculopapular drug rash. Common drugs causing urticaria are penicillin, NSAIDs, codeine and sulfonamides. It may also follow blood transfusion. Angioedema due to adverse effect of a drug is relatively uncommon and may be a complication of NSAIDs, angiotensin converting enzyme inhibitor (ACEI) therapy (captopril, enalapril maleate, lisinopril) and angiotensin receptor blocker (ARB) therapy. Among the ACEI users 0.1–0.7% develop angioedema and ACEIs are the precipitating cause in 17% of all hospital admissions due to angioedema. ARBs (mostly losartan) may induce angioedema in patients who had ACEI-induced angioedema earlier (32%). These drugs may also exacerbate pre-existing chronic idiopathic urticaria and/or angioedema.

Why the Disease is an Emergency?

• Drug-induced urticaria may be severe enough and sometimes it may be the presenting feature of drug-induced anaphylaxis or serum sickness like reactions.
• ACEIs may occasionally cause life-threatening angioedema resulting in laryngeal obstruction, and approximately 13 to 22% of these patients require airway interventions like endotracheal intubation and tracheostomy.
• ACEIs may rarely induce visceral angioedema, manifested as pain abdomen and vomiting, necessitating repeated hospital admission and surgical intervention. Clinicians must be aware of this complication of ACEI therapy.

Population at Risk

ACEI induced angioedema is more likely to occur if:
- Patient has previous history of angioedema,
- Patient suffers from hereditary angioedema,
- Patient has developed ACEI induced cough during therapy,
- Patients of afro-caribbean lineage,
- In female patients,
- Among smokers,
- Patients with perennial allergic disorders,
- Obese patients,
- Patients with sleep apnea.

Clinical Presentation

There is history of the drug intake followed by appearance of urticaria and/or angioedema. The involvement may be severe and there is no remission unless the culprit drug is withdrawn. In most patients (48–72%) on treatment with ACEI, angioedema may occur during first week of therapy; in others, the onset may be as late as 7 years after continuous therapy. Majority of the cases are milder and usually self-resolution occurs by 24 to 48 hours.

Clinical Clues

- There is temporal correlation between drug intake and occurrence of urticaria and/or angioedema.
- ACEI-induced angioedema is almost always without wheals and pruritus, affecting head, neck, oral mucosa and usually asymmetrical.
- In ACEI-induced angioedema usually patients are of older age group as compared to hereditary angioedema.

Differential Diagnosis

- Idiopathic urticaria and angioedema
- Hereditary angioedema.

Rapid Diagnostic Laboratory Method

- Increased level of CRP is a feature of ACEI-induced angioedema and may help to differentiate from other types of angioedema.
- In diagnostic confusion with hereditary angioedema, serum complement levels may be assessed, which are normal in ACEI-induced angioedema.
- Abdominal CT scan should be done in cases of suspected visceral angioedema induced by ACEI, which reveals thickened bowel wall and ascites. In case, oral contrast CT is done, the contrast media is visible

in the bowel lumen, surrounded by edematous bowel wall (target-sign appearance).

Management

Immediate withdrawal of the drug is mandatory. The management of drug induced urticaria and angioedema is similar to as ordinary urticaria and angioedema (discussed in subsequent section). ACEI-induced angioedema (bradykinin mediated) is almost always refractory to treatment with antihistamines, steroid and adrenaline. Following modalities have been tried in ACEI-induced angioedema:

- Fresh frozen plasma during an acute episode of laryngeal edema.
- In few studies, icatibant (bradykinin receptor 2 antagonist) has been observed to be effective in treating ACEI-induced angioedema. Single dose of subcutaneous injection of icatibant (30 mg) has been found to reduce the time for complete resolution of angioedema substantially and eliminates the need for invasive procedures to maintain upper airway patency. However, this mode of therapy requires further approval in larger studies.
- In patients of ACEI-induced angioedema, other ACEIs must be avoided (class effect). A different class of antihypertensive, preferably a calcium channel blocker may be used. ARBs must also be used with due care as cross sensitivity may occur.

Serum Sickness

Introduction

Serum sickness (SS) is a type III hypersensitivity reaction (immune complex mediated) occurring within 5 days to 3 weeks after exposure to a serum or other biological products. Among the biological products, important are IVIg, vaccines containing sera, streptokinase, antithymocyte globulin, antivenoms, polyclonal and monoclonal antibodies prepared from animal sera, etc. Some monoclonal antibodies causing SS are infliximab, rituximab and omalizumab. Hymenoptera stings (bees) may also cause serum sickness. Incidence of serum sickness is variable and depends upon the product used (chances are more with anti-rabies vaccine, as compared to tetanus toxoid).

Non-protein drugs may cause SS-like reactions. Important among these are aspirin, penicillin, cephalosporins (particularly cefaclor), sulphonamides, streptomycin, minocycline, ciprofloxacin, griseofulvin, etc. SS-like reactions differ from SS by lack of immune complex formation, hypocomplementemia, renal involvement and vasculitis.

Some cases of SS are mild and self-limiting; others may be associated with moderate to severe symptoms.

Why the Disease is an Emergency?

Usual time of occurrence of SS is by two weeks. However, in previously sensitized individuals, the onset may be stormy, within 12 to 36 hours of exposure.

SS may have any of the following acute presentations:
- Acute renal failure, which may be progressive leading to fatality.
- Neuropathy and other severe neurological complications.
- Gastrointestinal involvement manifested as pain abdomen, nausea, vomiting and diarrhea.
- Blurring of vision.
- Chest pain or breathlessness, resulting from pulmonary or cardiac involvement.
- Vasculitis.
- Shock.

Population at Risk

Antibiotic associated SS-like reactions are more common in children < 5 years.

Clinical Presentation

The commonest features of SS are fever, joint pain and urticarial wheals. Mild cases present with only these features. In cases with severe serum sickness, there is fever, urticaria and angioedema, arthritis, lymphadenopathy, glomerulonephritis, acute abdomen, pleuritis and endocarditis.

Clinical Clues

Clinical triad of fever, arthralgia and skin lesions within 2 weeks of using biological products in a patient should alert the treating physician of the possibility of SS. However, these clinical features may well resemble any other infectious illness and hence, it is difficult to diagnose unless this differential diagnosis is kept in mind. In the era of immunotherapy and biological therapy, SS must be kept as a diagnostic possibility.

Differential Diagnosis

- Urticaria and angioedema
- Drug-induced anaphylaxis
- Infections or autoimmune disorders presenting with fever, arthralgia and skin rash.

Rapid Diagnostic Laboratory Method

There is no test to confirm the diagnosis. Routine laboratory testing may reveal following:
- Raised ESR
- Elevated CRP

- Variable leukocyte count with or without eosinophilia
- Presence of plasma cells in peripheral blood smear
- Proteinuria/hematuria
- Transient elevation of serum creatinine
- Decreased serum complements (C3, C4).

Management

Mild cases of SS may be managed symptomatically. Patients with multisystem manifestations and acute presentation must be managed in an ICU. Patients with comorbid conditions/risk factors (immunocompromised state, extremes of age) must also be hospitalized. Immediate withdrawal of the causative agent is essential. Antihistamines, NSAIDs and systemic corticosteroids are the mainstay of management in mild/severe cases of SS.

ANAPHYLAXIS

Introduction

It is the IgE mediated type I hypersensitivity reaction induced by various agents, most commonly drugs, food allergens and bites/stings from venomous insects. Prevalence of anaphylaxis is around 2%.

Common drugs causing anaphylaxis are radiographic contrast media, antibiotics (penicillin), preparations containing animal sera, vaccines containing egg albumin, local and general anesthetics, etc. Anaphylaxis usually occurs during second exposure to a drug, but may also occur during the first exposure. The incidence of drug induced anaphylaxis is 1 in 5000 drug exposure and <10% cases are fatal (1in 50,000 to 1 in 100,000 patients treated with penicillin may develop anaphylaxis).

Why the Disease is an Emergency?

The onset and course of anaphylaxis is unpredictable, stormy and downhill. The clinician is usually unequipped with the armamentarium to manage anaphylaxis and the patient rapidly succumbs to hypotensive shock. Severity and fatality of anaphylaxis is directly proportional to the rapidity of its evolution. Death in anaphylaxis may occur due to respiratory obstruction or cardiovascular failure.

Population at Risk

Young and middle aged adults are more at risk to develop anaphylaxis. Susceptible people who have been advised the drug at intermittent schedule rather than continuous dosage and those who are receiving parenteral preparation rather than oral, are at higher risk to develop anaphylaxis. Symptoms are intensified in atopic individuals and in patients with cardiovascular compromise. Patients who are on treatment with β-blockers, ACEIs and ARBs, show blunted physiologic response and a poor outcome in anaphylaxis.

Clinical Presentation

There is acute onset of symptoms, within minutes to hours of the drug administration (mostly within 1 hour). Initially there is intense pruritus, urticaria and angioedema; thereafter, there is flushing (vasodilatation), headache, abdominal pain, vomiting and diarrhea (increased gastrointestinal motility), stridor (laryngeal edema), palpitation (tachycardia), hypotension and shock. In relatively milder cases, there may be premonitory symptoms like, dizziness, fainting attack, tingling sensation on skin and ocular erythema. Sometimes (20%), there may be a recurrence of symptoms after a gap of about 1 to 8 hours following subsidence of the initial episode (biphasic course).

Clinical Clues

Immediate onset of symptoms with drug administration should raise the suspicion of anaphylaxis. Both cutaneous and systemic symptoms are severe and there is dramatic progression. Every patient may not develop all features of anaphylaxis and incomplete features should not prevent a clinician to suspect anaphylaxis.

Rapid Laboratory Diagnostic Methods

Diagnosis of anaphylaxis is based on history and clinical features. There is no diagnostic test. **Table 2.3** presents various points to be asked about while eliciting history in a case of anaphylaxis.

Differential Diagnosis

- Anaphylactoid reaction; some of the drugs cause anaphylactoid reaction (clinical features similar to anaphylaxis but IgE independent) and these include NSAIDs, ciprofloxacin, mannitol, radiographic contrast media, etc.
- Severe acute urticaria and angioedema
- Vasovagal attack
- Acute episode of asthma leading to respiratory decompensation
- Foreign body aspiration.

Management

Anaphylaxis is an acute, life-threatening illness requiring immediate transportation to hospital (ICU) in an ambulance equipped with oxygen cylinder and other life saving instruments and trained health care personnel. Adrenaline is the drug of choice in the management of anaphylaxis.

Table 2.3: Details of history taking in a case of anaphylaxis

Information regarding symptoms during acute episode	• Flushing • Pruritus • Urticaria • Angioedema • Stridor and asphyxia • Abdominal colic • Vomiting and purging • Palpitation, constriction of chest • Syncope
Information regarding the agents encountered before onset of the symptoms	• Food intake (peanut, fish, egg, seafood, cow's milk) • Drug intake/administered • Blood transfusion • Insect bite/sting (bee/wasp) • Latex
Information regarding patient's activities preceding the episode	• Physical exercise • Sexual intercourse (semen)

- Supine position with elevation of lower limbs.
- Maintenance of airways and oxygen inhalation.
- First line treatment: Immediate administration of injection adrenaline (1:1000) solution, (0.01 mg/kg) maximum 0.5–1 ml, intramuscular on lateral aspect of thigh (larger surface area, faster absorption). The dose may be repeated every 5 to 20 minutes, if necessary.
- Intravenous fluid (normal saline/5% dextrose solution/colloidal volume expanders), particularly in patients with persistent hypotension in spite of adrenaline dosage.
- If there is no relief of symptoms of anaphylaxis with above treatment, adrenaline infusion may be instituted under the supervision of a physician experienced in continuous cardiovascular monitoring.
- If IM adrenaline and IV fluid replacement fail to correct hypotension, dopamine infusion may be started.
- In presence of bronchospasm; injection aminophylline 250 mg IV is administered over 5 minutes; thereafter it is continued as 250 mg by slow IV infusion (over 6 hours) mixed in 500 ml normal saline.
  OR
  Terbutaline/salbutamol nebulizer
- In presence of urticaria/angioedema/intense pruritus,
  Injection chlorpheniramine maleate (10–20 mg) administered IV
  OR
  Injection hydroxyzine 25 to 50 mg IM, thereafter 4 times daily, orally,
  OR
  Combination of H_1 and H_2 antihistamines

- Corticosteroids: Role of corticosteroid in the management of anaphylaxis is controversial as this has a slower onset of action. However, it may be helpful in protracted cases and in preventing the biphasic reaction. Following dose may be used:
  Injection hydrocortisone (250 mg) administered IV immediately, thereafter 100 mg 6 hourly. Once the patient is stabilized, oral prednisolone is started (40 mg/day for 3 days).
- All patients with an episode of anaphylaxis must be under supervision of the medical team for a minimum period of 4 to 6 hours or more to avoid the risk of biphasic reaction.
- All patients with one episode of anaphylaxis must be counseled thoroughly for avoidance of causative agent and must be provided with a medical information tag (bracelet/necklace/badge) with mention of anaphylaxis and its immediate management.

VASCULAR DISORDERS

A. Urticaria and angioedema
B. Purpura fulminans
C. Antiphospholipid antibody syndrome
D. Calciphylaxis
E. Kawasaki disease

Acute Urticaria and Angioedema

Introduction

Urticaria is a common dermatological illness of varied etiology, associated with sudden onset of intense pruritus and erythematous wheals. Urticaria may be 'acute onset', 'chronic' or 'acute on chronic.'

Angioedema is a common accompaniment of urticaria (50%), where there is diffuse edema of the involved body part or mucosa, and occasionally it may be fatal due to involvement of the pharyngeal/laryngeal mucosa.

Hereditary angioedema (HAE) is a rare autosomal dominant disorder, occurring due to hereditary deficiency or dysfunction of C1 esterase inhibitor, causing recurrent episodes of fatal angioedema. Acquired angioedema (AAE) is also a rare condition, where C1 esterase inhibitor deficiency is associated with B-cell lymphoproliferative disorder or autoimmune disorders (SLE) or due to presence of autoantibodies against this molecule. Drugs like ACEIs may also induce recurrent episodes of angioedema. These three types of angioedema are distinct from urticaria associated angioedema as the former conditions are mediated by the potent vasodilator bradykinin rather than histamine. In some cases of isolated angioedema, no underlying cause can be detected and these are designated as 'idiopathic angioedema.'

Not all episodes of urticaria and/or angioedema constitute an emergency situation, but patients with severe acute episodes with or without upper airway obstruction may present in the emergency room.

Why the Disease is an Emergency?

- A severe episode of acute urticaria may be quite distressing due to histamine mediated vasodilatation related symptoms, mostly flushing, intense pruritus and unsightly skin lesions.
- Urticaria and angioedema may present with visceral symptoms like acute pain abdomen. There may also be fatal pharyngeal and laryngeal edema resulting in obstruction and asphyxia.
- In hereditary angioedema, laryngeal obstruction leads to fatality in 2% cases, and in spite of receiving prophylactic treatment, 50% patients develop laryngeal edema. Acquired angioedema and ACEI-induced angioedema may also present with asphyxia.

Clinical Presentation

There is sudden appearance of erythematous wheals of varying size involving large body surface area, which may attain bizarre pattern due to confluence of the lesions (**Figure 2.6**). These are transient and resolution occurs within 24 hours (with/without treatment). There may be associated systemic symptoms like headache, fever, pain abdomen, vomiting and syncope.

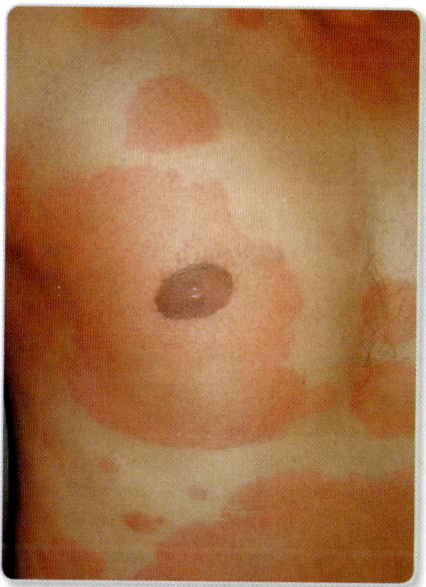

Figure 2.6: Acute urticaria

Angioedema presents as deep swelling involving face, lips, tongue or any other body part (**Figures 2.7A and B**). The swelling is non-pruritic but may be associated with pain. In hereditary angioedema and acquired angioedema the swelling typically appears over several hours and persists for next few days. These patients may also have severe abdominal pain and vomiting due to edema of the bowel wall and intestinal obstruction. Several family members may be affected in HAE.

Clinical Clues

- Transient, erythematous wheals associated with moderate to intense pruritus are indicative of urticaria.
- Diffuse and sometimes disfiguring edema around eyelids, lips, buccal mucosa, tongue or any other body part is suggestive of angioedema. Facial edema may be severe enough to obliterate the periorbital hollow and alter the facial contour. Late onset angioedema is usually acquired, whereas hereditary angioedema starts at early age.
- Recurrent long lasting angioedema, often unilateral, affecting several family members should point to the diagnosis of hereditary angioedema.
- Recent onset of recurrent episodes of angioedema in elderly hypertensive patient may be due to ACEI and drug history should be taken meticulously.

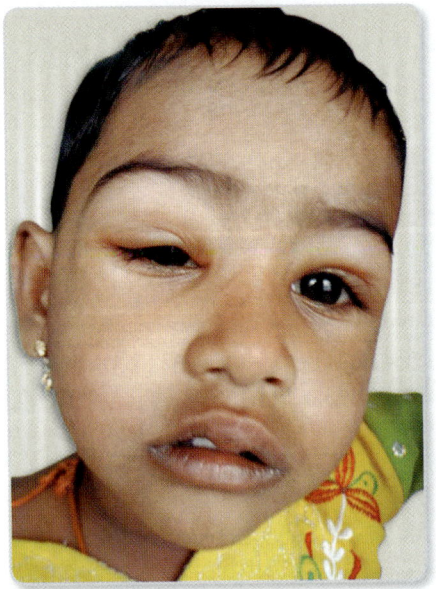

Figure 2.7A: Angioedema

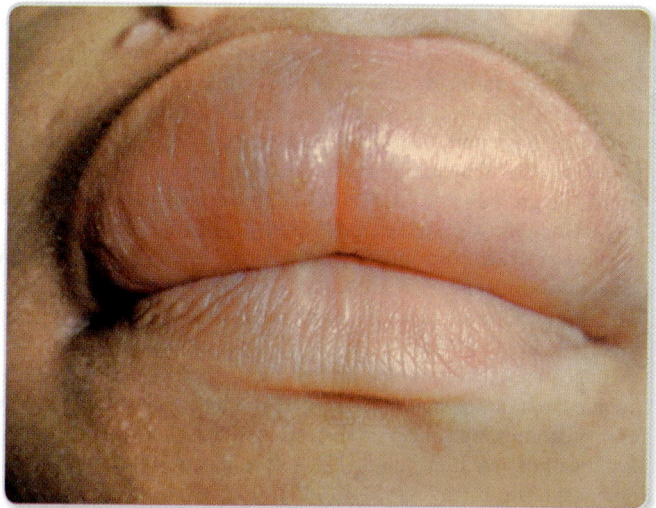

Figure 2.7B: Angioedema involving upper lip

Rapid Laboratory Diagnostic Methods

Routine investigations are unnecessary in patients presenting with acute urticaria and/or angioedema as these are non-contributory. If history of exposure to any specific allergen is given by the patient, investigations may be done once the acute episode is over (skin prick test/CAP fluoroimmunoassay, to measure allergen specific IgE). Prick test must be avoided if there is suspicion of anaphylaxis.

Patients with repeated episodes of angioedema and positive family history should be screened for hereditary angioedema (low plasma C4 and normal C3 is typical of HAE; low C1 inhibitor level, found in 85% patients makes definitive diagnosis of HAE; in 15% patients where C1 inhibitor level is normal or high, C1 inhibitor functional assay has to be done). Hereditary angioedema and acquired angioedema may be differentiated by C1q level, which is reduced in the latter.

Patients with acute-on-chronic urticaria must be worked up for any underlying cause during a period of remission.

Differential Diagnosis

- Drug-induced urticaria and angioedema.
- Anaphylaxis.
- Urticarial vasculitis (wheals are persistent > 24 hours, show an ecchymotic hue, may be tender and heals with hyperpigmentation. Systemic features may be marked).
- Systemic mastocytosis (visceral involvement including hematopoietic system).

Management

- In all patients with urticaria and angioedema, a thorough history of any precipitating factor (drug, food, food additives, heat, cold, physical exercise, etc.) must be elicited and is of immense importance in the management. Common precipitating factors for hereditary angioedema and acquired angiodema are *H. pylori* infection, stress, minor dental surgery, ACEI, oral contraceptive pill and hormone replacement therapy, which must be avoided in these patients.
- In all cases of urticaria and/or angioedema, any complaint of choking sensation, difficulty in swallowing or breathing should be attended with due importance as these may be early indicators of oropharyngeal involvement.
- Management algorithm for an episode of acute urticaria and/or angioedema has been presented in **Flow chart 1**. Second generation non-sedating antihistamines (levocetirizine, loratadine, desloratadine, fexofenadine, etc.) are the first line of management, and in case of non-response to standard dose, the dosage of these drugs may be hiked up to 4 times the usual (EAACI/GA(2)LEN/EDF/WAO guideline: management of urticaria, 2009).
- Any patient with angioedema presented with features of laryngeal obstruction must be intubated (or tracheostomy to be done) immediately.
- Hereditary angioedema and acquired angioedema do not respond to antihistamines and other mast cell inhibitors as bradykinin is the mediator in these conditions. Management of acute attack and prophylactic treatment of these conditions has been presented in flow chart 1. Prophylactic treatment of these patients is indicated if there is > 1 severe attack/month or before surgical procedures or during unavoidable stressful situation. All patients with acquired angioedema must be investigated for underlying disorder.
- Females with hereditary angioedema must avoid estrogen containing contraceptives. Acute episode of angioedema during pregnancy in these patients should be managed by replacement therapy with C1-inhibitor, and long-term prophylaxis may be achieved with transfusion of fresh frozen plasma or tranexamic acid.
- All patients with recurrent episodes of angioedema must be provided with a warning card to carry it along with them, depicting their diagnosis and management guidelines.

Purpura Fulminans

Introduction

Purpura fulminans (PF) is an acute onset fatal coagulation disorder characterized by progressive cutaneous hemorrhage, necrosis and disseminated intravascular coagulation (DIC), resulting from congenital or acquired deficiency of naturally occurring anticoagulants (protein C, protein S and/or antithrombin III).

Dermatological Emergencies

Flow chart 2.1: Management protocol in urticaria and angioedema

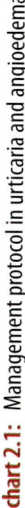

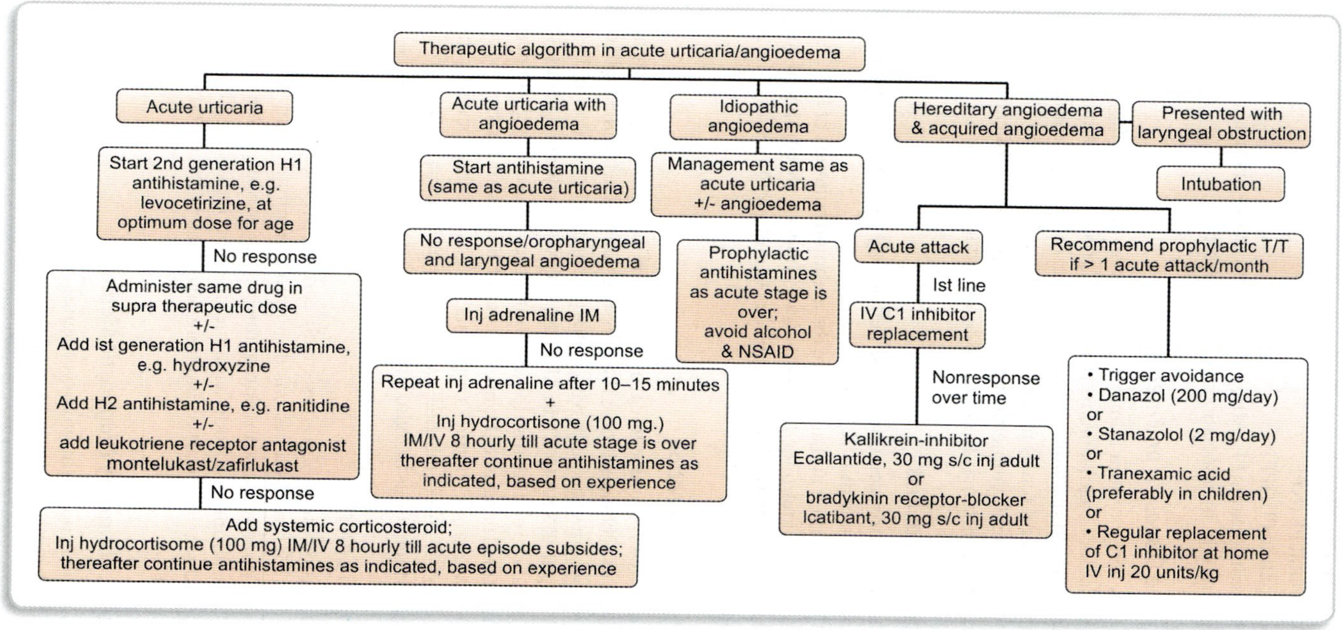

Therapeutic algorithm in acute urticaria/angioedema

- **Acute urticaria**
  - Start 2nd generation H1 antihistamine, e.g. levocetirizine, at optimum dose for age
  - No response
  - Administer same drug in supra therapeutic dose +/−
  - Add 1st generation H1 antihistamine, e.g. hydroxyzine +/−
  - Add H2 antihistamine, e.g. ranitidine +/−
  - add leukotriene receptor antagonist montelukast/zafirlukast
  - No response
  - Add systemic corticosteroid; Inj hydrocortisome (100 mg) IM/IV 8 hourly till acute episode subsides; thereafter continue antihistamines as indicated, based on experience

- **Acute urticaria with angioedema**
  - Start antihistamine (same as acute urticaria)
  - No response/oropharyngeal and laryngeal angioedema
  - Inj adrenaline IM
  - No response
  - Repeat inj adrenaline after 10–15 minutes +
  - Inj hydrocortisone (100 mg.) IM/IV 8 hourly till acute stage is over thereafter continue antihistamines as indicated, based on experience

- **Idiopathic angioedema**
  - Management same as acute urticaria +/− angioedema
  - Prophylactic antihistamines as acute stage is over; avoid alcohol & NSAID

- **Hereditary angioedema & acquired angioedema**
  - Acute attack
    - 1st line
    - IV C1 inhibitor replacement
    - Nonresponse over time
    - Kallikrein-inhibitor Ecallantide, 30 mg s/c inj adult or bradykinin receptor-blocker Icatibant, 30 mg s/c inj adult
  - Recommend prophylactic T/T if > 1 acute attack/month
    - Trigger avoidance
    - Danazol (200 mg/day) or
    - Stanazolol (2 mg/day) or
    - Tranexamic acid (preferably in children) or
    - Regular replacement of C1 inhibitor at home IV inj 20 units/kg

- **Presented with laryngeal obstruction**
  - Intubation

43

Three variants of the disease are:
- Neonatal PF (NPF)
- Idiopathic PF (IPF)
- Acute infectious PF (AIPF); this variant of the disease is encountered commonly, in association with septicemia.

Why the Disease is an Emergency?

Patients with purpura fulmimans are at risk of developing disseminated intravascular coagulation, resulting in hypotension, circulatory collapse, hypovolemic shock and multi-organ failure. Thrombotic episodes (cerebral, ophthalmic and renal) may occur in NPF and there may be blindness at birth. Peripheral symmetrical gangrene is a grave complication, especially with AIPF, which may lead to auto-amputation of digits.

Population at Risk

- NPF (homozygous protein C deficiency) may be present at birth or manifested within 72 hours.
- Older children and adults are the common sufferers of IPF.
- AIPF is commoner in infants and children as compared to adults because of lower baseline protein C and protein S level in this age group.

Clinical Presentation

Of the three variants, clinical picture of NPF is most severe. There are large patches of ecchymosis over the pressure points like buttocks and occiput, which becomes necrotic with a sharp demarcation line with the normal skin (**Figures 2.8A to C**). In AIPF the ecchymotic lesions are mostly over the distal extremities distributed symmetrically and may go for peripheral symmetrical gangrene (**Figure 2.9**). In IPF lesions are distributed centrally over lower trunk, buttocks, proximal thighs and legs, sparing the distal extremities. In established cases, there are widespread necrotic areas with erythematous margin, which may be topped with bullae.

Clinical Clues

Geographic areas of necrosis with narrow, livid, erythematous borders are the characteristic lesions of purpura fulminans with full evolution. Age of onset and distribution of the lesions provide a clue to the type of purpura fulminans. Underlying meningococcemia should be suspected if the skin lesions start as multiple petechiae with central dusky area of necrosis.

Rapid Laboratory Diagnostic Methods

- Platelet count (thrombocytopenia).
- Prothrombin time and partial thromboplastin time (prolonged).

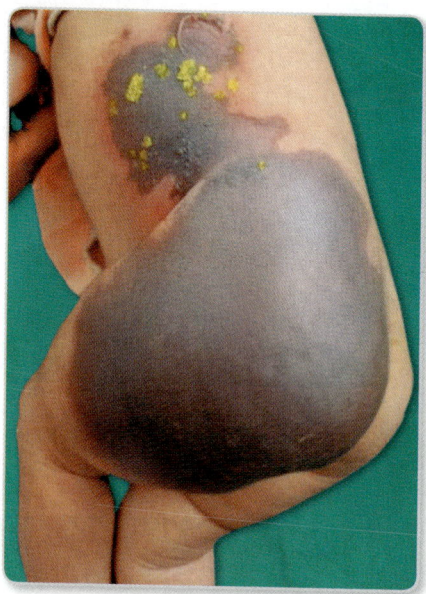

Figure 2.8A: Neonatal purpura fulminans

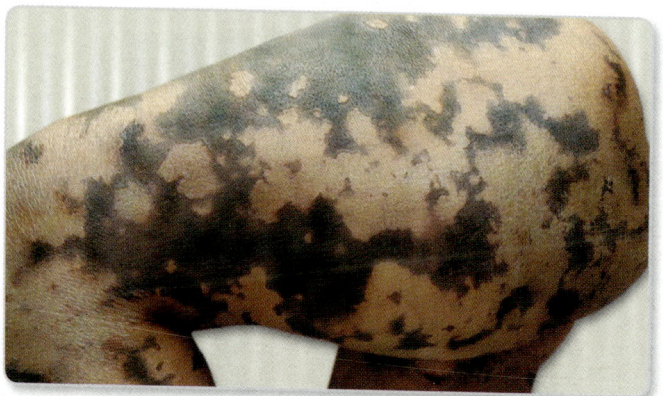

Figure 2.8B: Acute infectious purpura fulminans with geographic areas of cutaneous necrosis

- Fibrinogen and fibrin degradation product (decreased).
  The above three parameters may be normal initially; alteration is noted following appearance of skin lesions.
- D-dimer (positive), in initial phase of the disease, before appearance of skin lesions.

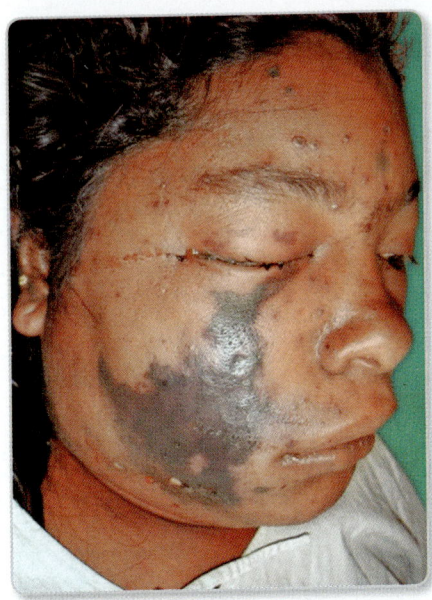

Figure 2.8C: Acute infectious purpura fulminans in a pregnant woman suffering from varicella

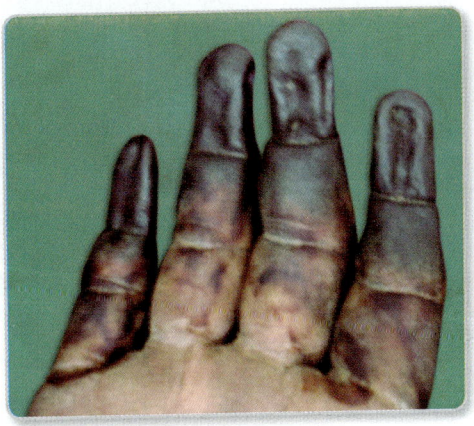

Figure 2.9: Peripheral symmetrical gangrene

- Blood culture/culture of other infective material to isolate the organism in case of AIPF.

Differential Diagnosis
- Cutaneous small vessel vasculitis.
- Thrombotic thrombocytopenic purpura.

- Antiphospholipid antibody syndrome.
- Warfarin and heparin induced cutaneous necrosis.

Management

- Treatment in an ICU is mandatory.
- Intravenous antibiotics according to culture/sensitivity report (AIPF).
- Fluid replacement and ventilatory support.
- Management of multi-organ failure.
- Treatment of NPF during acute and maintenance phase has been presented in **Table 2.4**. The mainstay of treatment in NPF is protein C concentrate replacement therapy. Anticoagulation with heparin (acute stage) followed by warfarin (chronic stage) is done with due care, as protein C deficient infants are susceptible to develop warfarin induced skin necrosis. These patients require lifelong anticoagulant therapy with prophylactic dose of protein C during invasive procedures.
- Surgical debridement as and when necessary.

Table 2.4: Treatment of neonatal purpura fulminans

Acute phase	• Fresh frozen plasma, 10–15 ml/kg, 8–12 hourly, till protein C is available/plasma protein C is >10 IU/dl. **Thereafter**, • Infusion of protein C concentrate (following test dose of 10U/kg), bolus dose 100U/kg, followed by 50 U/kg every 6 hourly, till plasma protein C is >50 IU/dl or normal circulating D-dimer + Unfractionated heparin 15–20 U/kg/hour, followed by low molecular weight heparin, 1–1.5 mg/kg, 12 hourly
Maintenance phase	• Infusion of protein C concentrate, 30–50 U/kg/1–3 days + Warfarin (0.05–0.1 mg/kg/day) OR • Warfarin alone (if protein C concentrate is not available)

Antiphospholipid Antibody Syndrome (Hughes Syndrome, Sneddon Syndrome)

Introduction

Persistent presence of antiphospholipid antibodies (lupus anticoagulant, anticardiolipin antibodies and anti-β-2-glycoprotein-1 antibody) in circulation resulting in symptom complexes of recurrent thromboembolic episodes and pregnancy loss is designated as antiphospholipid antibody syndrome (APLS). The prevalence of APLS is 1–5% among general population. APLS may be primary, secondary (associated with SLE, diabetes mellitus, various infections, malignancies, drugs, etc.) or catastrophic. Clinical features of APLS are highly variable, ranging from asymptomatic to recurrent, severe acute episodes.

Why the Disease is an Emergency?
- Thromboembolism in APLS may involve vital organs like heart, brain, liver (Budd-Chiari syndrome, risk <1%), kidney, etc.
- During pregnancy it may cause recurrent fetal loss. Preeclampsia/eclampsia and premature birth may occur (risk 10–20%).
- Catastrophic APLS, a rare variant, is associated with multi-organ thromboembolism and the mortality rate is as high as 50%.

Population at Risk
- Women are commonly affected; 75 to 90% of the patients with APLS are women.
- Patients with lupus (40–50%) may also suffer from APLS.

Clinical Presentation
The initial clinical presentation of patients with APLS may be venous thrombosis (hallmark feature), ischemic stroke or recurrent spontaneous abortions during pregnancy (hallmark feature). Thrombocytopenia may also be the presenting feature. Cutaneous features include:
- Livedo reticularis (frequent, > 20%)
- Livedoid vasculitis with painful leg ulcers (<10%)
- Splinter hemorrhage
- Cutaneous necrosis
- Digital gangrene [<10%] **(Figure 2.10)**.

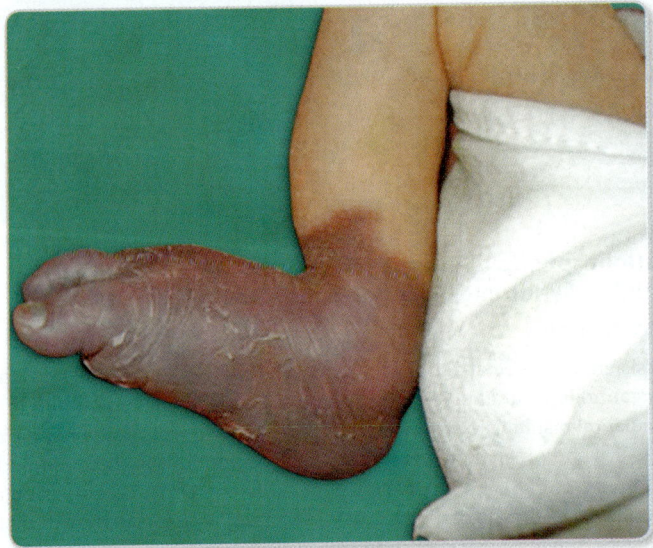

Figure 2.10: Gangrene of the foot in a neonate with antiphospholipid antibody syndrome

Clinical features arising from thrombotic episodes involving any viscera may be the presenting feature. Of thromboembolic episodes, deep vein thrombosis of lower limb is the commonest; others being pulmonary embolism and thrombosis involving portal vein, hepatic vein, mesenteric vein, splenic vein and cerebral vein (stroke/transient ischemic attack). Other neurological features include myelopathy, migraine and epilepsy. Valvular heart disease (mitral/aortic regurgitation) may be associated in 10 to 20% cases.

Clinical Clues

In a patient presenting with unexplained cutaneous necrosis or digital gangrene, history of recurrent thromboembolic episodes or recurrent, unexplained abortions (mostly in 2nd/3rd trimester) should raise the suspicion of APLS. In young patients with cerebrovascular accident, in absence of valvular heart disease, APLS must be ruled out.

In a patient with livedo reticularis and history of thrombosis, the clinician should suspect APLS and these patients are at high risk of arterial thrombosis.

Rapid Laboratory Diagnostic Methods

Diagnosis of APLS should be based on clinical and laboratory criteria. Among simple laboratory tests, platelet count may be done and presence of thrombocytopenia is a supportive feature. If facilities are available, following tests may be done:

- Anticardiolipin antibody; moderate to high level of (IgM/IgG), on two or more occasions at 12 weeks apart.
- Lupus anticoagulant antibodies; demonstrable on two or more occasions at 12 weeks apart.
- Imaging study (color Doppler, CT scan, MRI scan) of the vascular system/organ affected by thrombosis

Differential Diagnosis

- Thrombotic, thrombocytopenic purpura
- Disseminated intravascular coagulation
- Heparin-induced thrombocytopenia syndrome
- Hemolytic uremic syndrome.

Management

Management of APLS requires multi-specialty approach. Mainstay of treatment is anticoagulant therapy. Dermatologists' consultation is asked for in presence of cutaneous involvement. Decision of anticoagulant therapy depends upon the extent of the disease. Following is a brief guideline regarding treatment of APLS.

- In presence of thrombosis (arterial/venous), anticoagulation with warfarin must be done (INR to be maintained between 2.0–3.0).

- In patients with recurrent thrombosis, low dose aspirin (81 mg/day) has to be added to warfarin (INR 3.0–4.0).
- Management during pregnancy:
  - For asymptomatic antiphospholipid antibody positivity during pregnancy and for single pregnancy loss (<10 weeks), no active treatment is required.
  - In case of recurrent pregnancy loss (<10 weeks/> 10 weeks), without history of thrombosis, prophylactic dose of heparin (30–40 mg subcutaneously, OD) has to be given during pregnancy with low dose aspirin. During post partum period, these patients are to be treated with heparin up to 6 to 12 weeks, and thereafter with low dose aspirin.
  - In presence of recurrent fetal loss along with recurrent thrombosis during pregnancy, therapeutic dose of heparin (1 mg/kg subcutaneously BD OR 1.5 mg/kg subcutaneously, OD) has to be used along with low dose aspirin and warfarin during postpartum period.
- In case of catastrophic APLS, systemic corticosteroid and IVIg has to be added.
- Cutaneous necrosis is treated by symptomatic wound care. Digital gangrene may require amputation.

Calciphylaxis

Introduction

Calciphylaxis (calcific uremic arteriopathy) is a condition associated with chronic renal failure (CRF). There is arterial calcification resulting in complete vascular occlusion and cutaneous necrosis.

Why the Disease is an Emergency?

- Sepsis is the principal cause of death in patients with calciphylaxis.

Population at Risk

Patients with terminal CRF, especially if there is underlying hyperparathyroidism, are at risk to develop calciphylaxis. Women are more commonly affected.

Clinical Presentation

The initial lesion is a small, erythematous, tender area or widespread area of livedo reticularis, which rapidly progresses to intense erythema, induration and necrosis. The commonly involved sites are abdomen and proximal extremities (buttocks and thighs).

Clinical Clues

A rapidly progressing tender, erythematous plaque developing over abdomen and proximal extremities, in a patient with CRF should raise the suspicion of calcific uremic arteriopathy.

Rapid Laboratory Diagnostic Methods
- Blood urea/serum creatinine.
- Serum calcium and phosphorus.
- Imaging studies to identify vascular involvement.

Differential Diagnosis
The condition may simulate various other conditions:
- Peripheral arterial occlusive disease
- Infections (cellulitis/erysipelas, necrotizing fasciitis)
- Cryoglobulinemic vasculitis
- Panniculitis
- Coagulopathy (thromboembolism, disseminated intravascular coagulation, antiphospholipid antibody syndrome)

Management
As the affected patients are in advanced stage of CRF, there is poor response to therapy. Management requires a multi-disciplinary approach principally by a nephrologist. The hypercoagulable state of the patient requires careful monitoring and adjustment of anticoagulant dosage. General measures include:
- Maintenance of tissue perfusion by preventing hypotension.
- Correction of anemia and provision of optimum nutrition.
- Hyperbaric oxygen therapy.
- Maintenance of calcium homeostasis to prevent a hypercalcemic state (adjustment of the dialysate fluid, minimize vitamin D intake).
- Dialysis.
- Parathyroidectomy (in presence of hyperparathyroidism).
- Prevention of sepsis.
- Analgesics to relieve pain.
- Care of wound with debridement of the necrotic tissue.

Kawasaki Disease
(Mucocutaneous Lymph Node Syndrome)
Introduction
It is a febrile exanthematous illness affecting children, probably mediated by bacterial superantigen, causing multi-system vasculitis with predominant involvement of the coronary vessels. The disease has a worldwide prevalence with highest risk among Asians.

Why the Disease is an Emergency?
- During the acute phase of the disease, there is myocarditis resulting in arrhythmias and sudden death due to myocardial infarction.
- Subsequently (subacute stage), multiple coronary aneurysms may develop (25% cases) and there are risks of thromboembolism, coronary occlusion, ruptured aneurysms and sudden death.

- Thrombotic episodes may involve other organs.
- Gangrene of lower limbs and DIC may occur rarely.

Population at Risk

Children, often < 2 years are the common sufferers of Kawasaki disease. Male children are more commonly affected. Age < 1 year is a poor prognostic factor.

Clinical Presentation

There is acute onset high fever persisting for 5 to 7 days, associated with mucosal and conjunctival congestion. The child is extremely irritable. A generalized, faint maculopapular rash appears on 3rd/4th day and later localized to distal extremities. The illness remits with periungual desquamation after 1 to 3 weeks of onset. Cervical lymphadenopathy and edema of hands and feet are the other features. Systemic involvement includes arthritis, myocarditis, nephritis and meningitis. The disease has been divided into three phases:
- Acute febrile phase.
- Subacute phase (up to 4th week after the onset of illness), when fever is subsided but irritability, anorexia and conjunctivitis persists. Coronary aneurysm may form, and risk of sudden death is highest at this time.
- Convalescent phase (usually 6 to 8 weeks after onset of illness); there is no sign or symptom of illness at this phase and convalescence is considered till ESR returns to normal.

Diagnostic criteria for Kawasaki disease are available. However, incomplete form of the disease may occur.

Clinical Clues

In a febrile child (fever > 104°F, for > 5 days), not responding to therapy, following clinical features should prompt the clinician to make a diagnosis of Kawasaki disease:
- Strawberry tongue and fissured lips (**Figure 2.11A**).
- Nonpurulent conjunctivitis with perilimbal sparing and without tearing.
- Cervical lymphadenopathy (usually unilateral, > 1.5 cm in size).
- Perineal desquamating rash in acute stage (**Figure 2.11B**).
- Myocarditis.
- Periungual desquamation, when the febrile episode subsides (**Figure 2.11C**).

Rapid Laboratory Diagnostic Methods

Kawasaki disease is a clinical diagnosis, and no laboratory test is diagnostic of this condition. Routine laboratory tests reveal:
- Low hemoglobin.*
- Leukocytosis with large number of immature cells (band cells).*

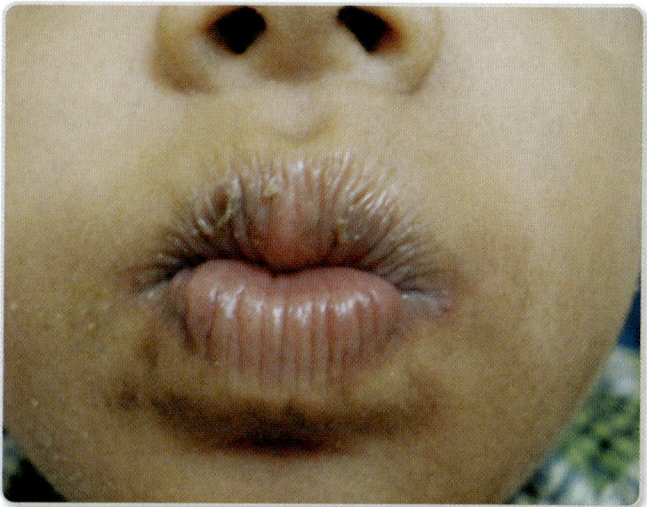

Figure 2.11A: Fissured lips in a child with Kawasaki disease

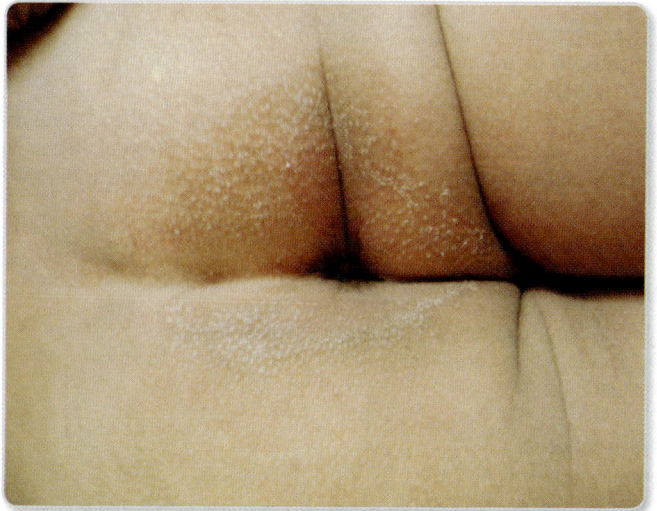

Figure 2.11B: Perianal desquamation in a child with Kawasaki disease

- Elevated ESR.
- Thrombocytosis (in the subacute phase).
- Thrombocytopenia.*
- Low albumin and low serum IgG (age adjusted).*
- High CRP.

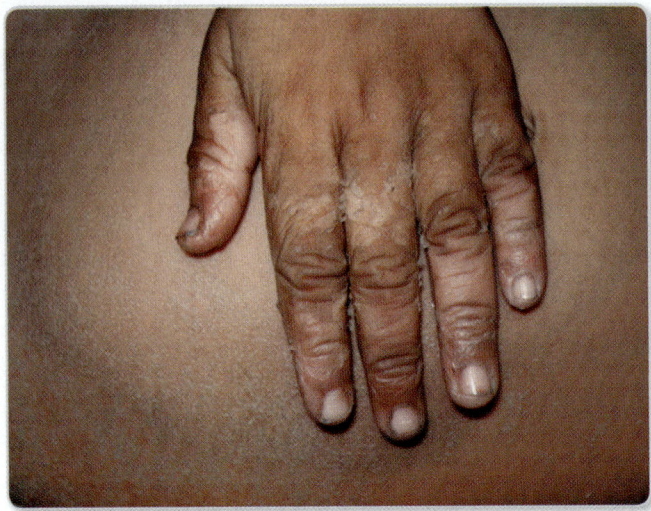

Figure 2.11C: Periungual desquamation in a child with Kawasaki disease

- Sterile pyuria.
- Raised liver enzymes.*
- ECG (myocarditis).
- Echocardiography (to rule out myocarditis and coronary aneurysm); to be done routinely at diagnosis and after 2 to 3 weeks of illness. If no abnormality is found on these two occasions, it is repeated at 6 to 8 week or at the normalization of ESR.

*Predictors of more severe outcome

Differential Diagnosis

- Viral exanthematous illnesses, particularly measles.
- Maculopapular drug rash.
- Scarlet fever.

Management

Acute phase:
- Single high dose IVIg (2g/kg) infusion over 10 to 12 hours,

+

- Aspirin, 80 to 100 mg/kg/day, 6 hourly divided doses till 14th day.

IVIg + aspirin (if administered within initial 10 days) decrease the occurrence of coronary artery disease.

If there is no/partial response to initial single dose of IVIg, additional 1 dose may be administered.

Convalescent phase:
- Aspirin 35 mg/kg OD, till 6 to 8 weeks after onset of illness.
- Follow-up screening for development of coronary complications. Patients with coronary artery involvement should receive long term therapy with aspirin, dipyridamole ± warfarin under the supervision of a cardiologist.
- Management of acute coronary thrombosis, if any.
- Long-term management of cardiovascular complications.

Role of corticosteroid in the treatment of Kawasaki disease is controversial. However, it may be used for patients with persistent fever, even after administration of 2 doses of IVIg.

COLLAGEN VASCULAR DISORDERS

Acute Cutaneous Lupus Erythematosus

Introduction

Acute cutaneous lupus erythematosus (ACLE) may be localized or generalized (Gilliam classification) and may occur as initial manifestation or as acute flare up in a case of systemic lupus erythematosus (SLE). In latter case, the course of ACLE may be waxing and waning depending on the severity of systemic disease.

Why the Disease is an Emergency?

Patients with acute cutaneous lupus erythematosus may have severe cutaneous involvement. The localized variant may present with disfiguring facial erythema and edema. In presence of underlying systemic lupus erythematosus, advanced internal organ involvement (pulmonary, renal) may be present.

Population at Risk

Patients suffering from systemic lupus erythematosus are at risk of developing bouts of ACLE, especially after unprotected exposure to sunlight or other UV-light source.

Patients with initial presentation as ACLE, run a higher risk of developing severe disease.

Clinical Presentation

Localized ACLE presents with typical, erythematous, edematous butterfly rash, extending centrally over nasal bridge and laterally to ear lobules (**Figure 2.12**). The forehead and 'V' area of neck is also involved. The lips may be swollen and covered with hemorrhagic crust.

Patients with generalized ACLE, in addition to the above features, develop a widespread morbilliform rash. In a hyperacute form of the

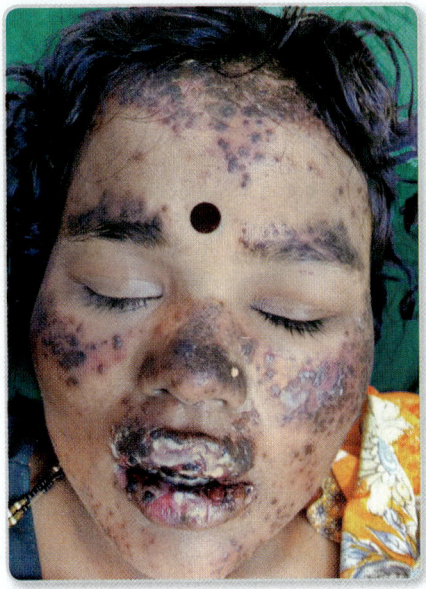

Figure 2.12: Acute cutaneous lupus erythematosus

disease, the rash may be vesiculo-bullous, simulating Stevens-Johnson syndrome/toxic epidermal necrolysis.

In both the forms severe photosensitivity may be associated. The condition is short-lasting and on adequate management, healing occurs rapidly with post-inflammatory hyperpigmentation but no scarring.

Clinical Clues

Typical sparing of the nasolabial folds is a characteristic feature of ACLE and helps in differentiating from other similar-looking conditions.

Rapid Laboratory Diagnostic Methods

There is no specific laboratory finding in ACLE. In all suspected cases, laboratory tests for collagen vascular disorders (antinuclear antibody, anti ds-DNA antibody) must be done to differentiate from other conditions. ESR and CRP indicates disease activity. Histopathologically, the prominent features are focal basal cell degeneration and upper dermal edema.

Lesional lupus band test may be positive.

In all patients with initial presentation as ACLE, screening for systemic involvement is mandatory (chest X-ray, urinalysis, renal function test, etc.).

Differential Diagnosis
- Dermatomyositis
- Rosacea
- Stevens-Johnson syndrome/toxic epidermal necrolysis.

Management
Patients with ACLE requires hospitalization:
- Rest in a relatively darker room.
- Anxiolytic.
- Systemic corticosteroids (0.5–1 mg/kg body weight).
- Other immunosuppressive drugs (cyclophosphamide/azathioprine) in presence of systemic involvement.
- Hydroxychloroquine (6.5 mg/kg/day) may be started as a future steroid-sparing agent.
- During healing, mild topical corticosteroid and/or topical tacrolimus/pimecrolimus may be added to hasten the recovery.
- Sunscreen as soon as the acute skin lesions subside.

COMPLICATED VASCULAR TUMORS
A. Kassabach Merritt syndrome
B. Multifocal/diffuse neonatal hemangiomatosis

A. Kassabach Merritt Syndrome
Introduction
It is a complication of tufted hemangioma and Kaposiform hemangioendothelioma (located in skin or other organ), wherein there is consumptive coagulopathy, thrombocytopenia and microangiopathic hemolytic anemia. The phenomenon is initiated inside the vascular tumor itself resulting in rapid increase in its size. The coagulopathy is long-standing but resolves spontaneously over several years (1–6 years) and the tumor becomes smaller and fibrotic.

Why the Disease is an Emergency?
Consumptive coagulopathy and thrombocytopenia leads to bleeding from various sites and the associated mortality is as high as 20 to 40%.

Population at Risk
Infants with these tumors, during the first few weeks of life; occurs rarely in adults.

Clinical Presentation
It may start at a vascular tumor at birth or anytime during infancy. There is sudden enlargement of the size of the lesion which becomes turgid

and bluish in color, looking almost cellulitic. There may be bleeding from other body sites, like epistaxis, hematuria and traumatic bleeding.

Clinical Clues

Sudden increase in the size of the vascular tumor (which becomes woody hard and ecchymotic), spreading beyond the borders of the lesion, along with multiple ecchymosis all over body and bleeding from various sites are the clinical pointers to the diagnosis.

Rapid Laboratory Diagnostic Methods

- Platelet count (thrombocytopenia); May decrease to <5000/mm^3. There may be a marginal decrease in platelet count initially, misleading the clinician.
- Coagulation profile (fibrinogen level, prothrombin time, activated partial prothrombin time, positive D-dimer).
- Reticulocyte count (increased in presence of hemolytic anemia).

Management

All episodes do not warrant energetic treatment as the coagulopathy may be mild and spontaneous resolution may occur. Regular monitoring of the child is necessary by estimating:
- Platelet count
- Coagulation profile
- Fibrinogen and D-dimer

In presence of severe consumptive coagulopathy, the infant must be managed in neonatal ICU. Treatment includes:
- Oral corticosteroids, prednisolone 2 to 5 mg/kg/day; (to reduce the bulk of the tumor, also beneficial by raising the platelet count). Less effective in presence of severe consumptive coagulopathy.
- Combination therapy (steroid and radiation therapy).
- Interferon α: administered subcutaneously (1–3 million units/m^2 of BSA/day) in children > 1 year. It inhibits angiogenesis inside the tumor and is slow acting (not a treatment of choice in presence of extensive coagulopathy).
- Vincristine (1–1.5 mg/m^2 of BSA/week by slow IV infusion × 12 weeks), given in children > 1 year. It acts by binding to platelets and is the most promising medical treatment following oral steroid. Response is evident by 4 weeks.
- Antiplatelet agents like aspirin, ticlopidine and dipyridamole.
- Surgical excision of small accessible tumors with or without preoperative tumor embolization.
- Antifibrinolytic agents like tranexamic acid and ε-aminocaproic acid.
- Transfusion: Platelet concentrate or fresh frozen plasma administered only during acute blood loss or operative procedures.

Multifocal/Diffuse Neonatal Hemangiomatosis

Introduction

This is a rare fatal disorder during infancy characterized by multiple visceral and cutaneous hemangiomas. Diagnosis requires presence of three criteria:
- Neonatal onset
- Involvement of ≥3 organs
- No malignant transformation.

Liver, lungs, gastrointestinal tract and brain are frequently involved.

Why the Disease is an Emergency?

It is associated with high mortality due to congestive cardiac failure (commonest), hemorrhage and multi-organ failure. Presence of heart failure and ≥ 5 organ involvement are poor prognostic indicators.

Population at Risk

Infants with numerous cutaneous and/or visceral hemangiomas.

Clinical Presentation

Multiple hemangiomas of skin are present at birth or appearing soon thereafter associated with hepatomegaly (due to visceral hemangioma) and/or evidence of gastrointestinal bleeding.

Clinical Clues

In a patient with multifocal cutaneous hemangioma, progressive increase in abdominal girth should raise the suspicion of diffuse hepatic hemangiomatosis and related risk of heart failure. Presence of ≥ 5 hemangiomas in an infant is an indication of screening for visceral hemangioma.

Rapid Laboratory Diagnostic Methods

- Stool for occult blood.
- Urine microscopy for presence of RBCs.

Imaging of internal organs to detect hemangiomas:
- Ultrasonography of liver.
- CT scan of lungs, brain and abdomen.

Management

The infant must be managed in neonatal ICU.
- First line of therapy: Oral corticosteroids, prednisolone 2 to 5 mg/kg/day; if no improvement is seen by 2 to 4 weeks, second line drug has to be added.

- Second line therapy: Interferon alpha; administered subcutaneously (1–3 million units/m^2 of BSA/day).
- Management of congestive cardiac failure.
- Surgical management for very large hepatic hemangioma (ligation of hepatic artery or embolization).

VESICULOBULLOUS DISORDERS

A. Genetic blistering disorders
B. Immunobullous disorder

Genetic Blistering Disorders

Introduction

Among the genetic blistering diseases, epidermolysis bullosa (EB) group of disorders present with skin fragility induced by even mild trauma. These disorders are rare and are of varying severity. There is defect in various components of the dermoepidermal junction, leading to skin fragility. Patients usually present at or soon after birth with multiple vesiculobullous lesions and widespread areas of erosions. There are several variants of epidermolysis bullosa, of which more severe forms are:

- Epidermolysis bullosa simplex (Dowling Meara variant).
- Junctional EB (Herlitz type).
- Autosomal recessive dystrophic EB (ARDEB).

Why the Disease is an Emergency?

- All patients with epidermolysis bullosa with extensive cutaneous involvement may develop features of acute skin failure due to loss of epidermal barrier. These patients are at increased risk of fatal infection and septicemia, spreading from skin lesions.
- Children with junctional EB (Herlitz type) may present with stridor due to supraglottic stenosis or laryngeal stricture and acute urinary retention due to urethral meatal stenosis.
- Patients with ARDEB presents with severe progressive esophageal stricture due to mucosal blistering starting during infancy, resulting in acute pain, dysphagia and partial or complete obstruction.
- Children with ARDEB may present with acute abdomen due to fecal retention as a sequelae of perianal erosions and anal fissure. There may also be acute urinary retention due to urethral meatal stenosis.
- Variants of EB simplex and junctional EB may be associated with pyloric atresia and these infants present with projectile vomiting soon after birth.

Clinical Presentation

- All patients with EB presents with spontaneous/minimal trauma-induced blistering over friction-prone body areas present at/soon after birth (**Figure 2.13**).
- There are widespread areas of denudation in some variants with scarring and/or milia formation.
- Involvement of teeth, nails and scarring alopecia are features of various forms of epidermolysis bullosa.

Clinical Clues

- Grouped blisters on erythematous base is a feature of EB simplex (Dowling Meara variant).
- Widespread blistering starting soon after birth, which heals slowly with atrophic scarring, hoarseness of voice and stridor are the clinical pointers to the diagnosis of junctional EB, Herlitz type. Older infants develop perioral and perinasal crusted erosions with exuberant granulation tissue characteristic of this disorder. Fingertips attain typical bulbous appearance with shedding of nails and formation of granulation tissue over nail bed and nail folds.
- Scarring and milia are characteristic cutaneous features of ARDEB. Other distinct features of this variant of the disease are scarring alopecia, microstomia, ankyloglossia and mitten deformity of hands and feet.

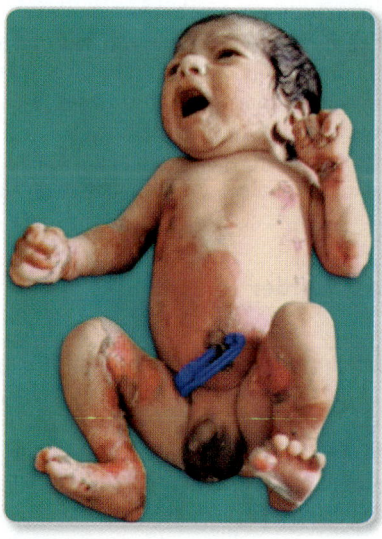

Figure 2.13: Widespread denudation of skin over trauma-prone body parts in a neonate with epidermolysis bullosa

Rapid Laboratory Diagnostic Methods

There is no specific rapid diagnostic method for epidermolysis bullosa. Tzanck smear should be done to rule out immunobullous disorders and staphylococcal scalded skin syndrome. If the lesions are infected, culture sensitivity test from lesional discharge should be done to select the antibiotics. If patient presents with septicemia, complete blood count, and blood culture is to be done.

Differential Diagnosis

- Immunobullous disorders
- Staphylococcal scalded skin syndrome

Management

Management of patients with severe forms of epidermolysis bullosa requires multidisciplinary approach.

It is preferable to constitute a specifically trained and dedicated team including clinicians from various specialties and nursing staffs to manage such patients. There is no specific treatment for this disorder and symptomatic management is important.

- Wound care is of utmost importance. Various artificial and biological dressing materials are commercially available for this purpose.
- Prevention of mildest trauma to protect from formation of fresh lesions. During dressing, adhesive tapes must be avoided in these patients. The health care providers and the mother must be trained specifically to handle the affected infant.
- If the patient presents with dysphagia and/or stridor, it should be managed immediately with the help of gastroenterologist/otorhinolaryngologist. Intestinal obstruction and acute urinary retention should also be managed accordingly.
- If the patient presents with acute skin failure due to widespread loss of skin, and related complications, it should be managed accordingly in a DICU.

Immunobullous Disorder

Introduction

The main disorders included in this group, which may present in the emergency room are pemphigus and bullous pemphigoid.

Why the Disease is an Emergency?

Patients with immunobullous disorders present with widespread areas of skin loss (erosions) leading to disruption of cutaneous barrier function. This may lead to acute skin failure with related complications like fluid and electrolyte imbalance, disturbed thermoregulation leading to hypothermia, septicemia, etc. Patients with pemphigus foliaceus may present with erythroderma and related complications.

Population at Risk

- Though it may occur at any age, young adults are the common sufferers of pemphigus.
- Elderly patients (> 60 years) are the common sufferers of bullous pemphigoid.

Clinical Presentation

- In patients with pemphigus vulgaris, the lesions may be localized (scalp/oral mucosa) in the initial period or severe and generalized from the beginning. There are large flaccid bullae which rupture to form large areas of erosions. Oral, pharyngeal or genital mucosae may be involved and there are painful erosions. The lesions heal without scarring but with post-inflammatory hyperpigmentation. In patients with pemphigus foliaceus, intact vesicles may not be seen as lesions are very transient and there may be diffuse scaling giving rise to erythroderma **(Figure 2.14A)**. Photosensitivity and localization of the lesions over butterfly area of face is the presenting feature of pemphigus erythematosus.

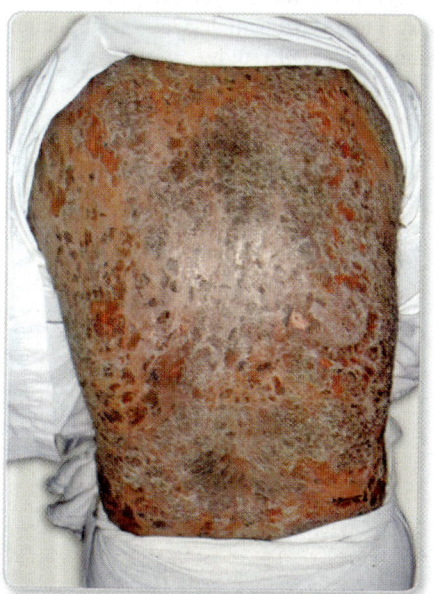

Figure 2.14A: Pemphigus foliaceus presenting as erythroderma

- In bullous pemphigoid, elderly people are the common sufferers. The patients present with pruritic urticarial wheals for few days (premonitory symptom) followed by appearance of tense bullae over the wheals. The bullae are persistent for few days, become hemorrhagic and heal with scarring, pigmentation and milia formation. Mucosal sites are rarely involved.

Clinical Clues

- Flaccid bullae arising on normal appearing skin with mucosal erosions are the characteristic lesions of pemphigus (**Figure 2.14B**).
- Tense hemorrhagic bullae arising on the background of urticarial lesions with or without scarring and milia formation are characteristic features of bullous pemphigoid (**Figures 2.15A and B**). Mucosal involvement may or may not be present.
- Nikolsky's sign and bulla spread sign are positive in pemphigus and is an important differentiating point from bullous pemphigoid.

Rapid Laboratory Diagnostic Methods

Laboratory tests for diagnostic purpose:
- Tzanck smear to demonstrate acantholytic cells is a reliable side laboratory technique to prove the diagnosis of pemphigus and negative Tzanck smear in the background of characteristic clinical features is suggestive of bullous pemphigoid.
- Skin biopsy for histopathological examination and direct immunofluorescence (DIF) study.

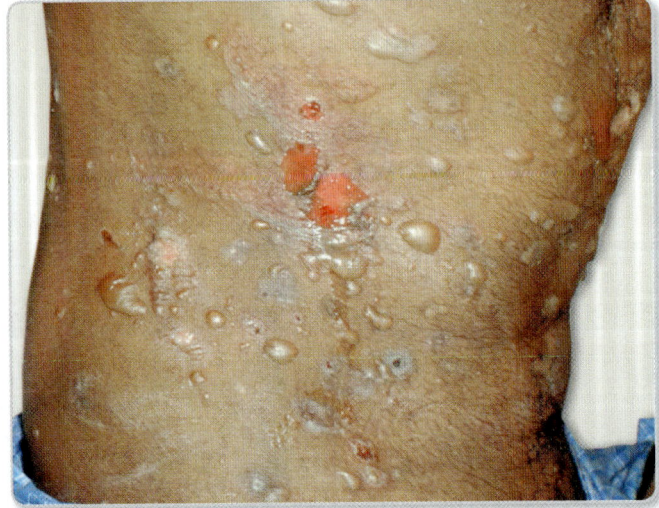

Figure 2.14B: Pemphigus vulgaris

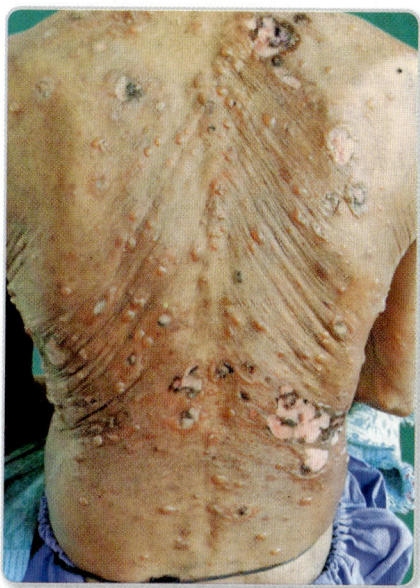

Figure 2.15A: Bullous pemphigoid

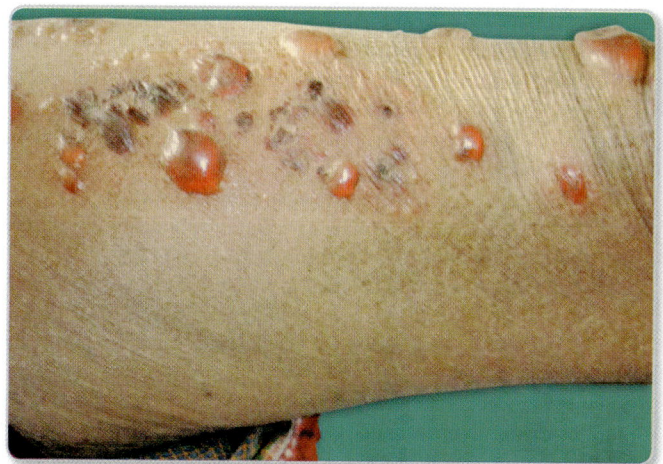

Figure 2.15B: Tense hemorrhagic bullae of bullous pemphigoid

Laboratory tests to be done in presence of acute skin failure:
- Complete hemogram.
- Serum electrolytes.
- Serum urea/creatinine.

- Repeated culture/sensitivity test from eroded skin.
- Blood sugar, especially in elderly patients.
- In all elderly patients with pemphigus and bullous pemphigoid, screening tests for underlying internal malignancy must be performed.

Differential Diagnosis

Pemphigus: Staphylococcal scalded skin syndrome, Stevens-Johnson syndrome, bullous pemphigoid.

Bullous pemphigoid: Pemphigus, Linear IgA disease, Stevens-Johnson syndrome.

Management

Patients with immunobullous disorders may present with acute skin failure and must be managed in DICU. The management protocol for these patients includes:

- Optimum environmental temperature to prevent hypothermia.
- Barrier nursing.
- Intravenous line (preferably through uninvolved skin).
- Urinary catheterization.
- Maintenance of fluid and electrolyte balance (intake/output chart).
- Intravenous antibiotics guided by culture/sensitivity report.
- Oral and ophthalmic care.
- Skin care:
  - Regular bath with an antibacterial soap (triclosan) or sponging (if the patient is not ambulant).
  - Drainage of fluid from large bullae and the blister roof is allowed to rest on the base as a natural dressing.
  - Large erosions are cleaned daily and covered with sterile paraffin-soaked gauze.
  - Nonsticky cotton clothing and bed clothes (McIntosh).
  - GV lotion (1%) may be applied over large erosions and apposing surfaces (e.g. genitalia, axillae, groin).
  - Adhesive tapes must be avoided in patients with pemphigus and roller bandage should be used instead.
- Diet rich in protein (liquid/bland semisolid, in presence of severe oral involvement.
- Supplementation of vitamins.
- Frequent change of posture in case of nonambulant patients and early ambulation.

Specific therapy includes:

Pemphigus: High dose parenteral systemic corticosteroid, preferably with immunosuppressive drugs (adjuvant therapy) at daily dosage or as monthly pulse therapy.

For patients with BP presented with extensive lesions, intravenous systemic corticosteroid (0.75–1 mg/kg) may be started to overcome the crisis, which can be tapered thereof to a minimum required dose and other drugs like dapsone/tetracyclines/mycophenolate mofetil are added for long-term remission.

INFECTIONS

A. Necrotizing fasciitis.
B. Meningococcemia.
C. Disseminated gonococcal infection.
D. Rocky Mountain spotted fever.
E. Dengue hemorrhagic fever.

Necrotizing Fasciitis

Introduction

Necrotizing fasciitis (NF) is a rare subcutaneous infection which spreads along the fascial plane and involves the muscular fascia and aponeurosis. There is an initial focus of infection, which may be subtle like minor abrasion, injection prick (drug addict), pyoderma, Bartholin's abscess (perineal NF), or complicated cases of erysipelas or cellulitis. Organisms are varied, commoner being *Streptococcus* or *Staphylococcus*; coliforms and anaerobic organisms may also cause NF. The infection may be monomicrobial or polymicrobial.

Why the Disease is an Emergency?

NF is associated with severe local and systemic complications and this is a life-threatening condition. The complications of NF include:
- Local complication: Deeper infection (myositis, pyomyositis); superficial extensive tissue damage due to sloughing results in mutilation which is difficult to manage.
- Systemic complications due to septicemia; fever, altered mental status, thrombocytopenia, hypotension and multi-organ failure.

Population at Risk

Malnourished children, patients with diabetes, alcoholism, venous incompetence, immunosuppression due to any cause. Wounds of varicella in children are a risk factor for development of NF and usually such infection is monomicrobial (group A β-hemolytic streptococcus), whereas traumatic wounds usually result in polymicrobial infection.

Clinical Presentation

Extremities and perineum are the common sites involved.

Patient presents with an area of inflammation simulating cellulitis, which progresses very fast. The patient is febrile with severe constitutional symptoms. The involved body part is edematous, hard, with alteration of color on the surface and loss of sensation. Gangrenous changes supervene (**Figures 2.16A and B**). As the disease progresses, features of systemic toxicity like high fever, disorientation and lethargy may supervene.

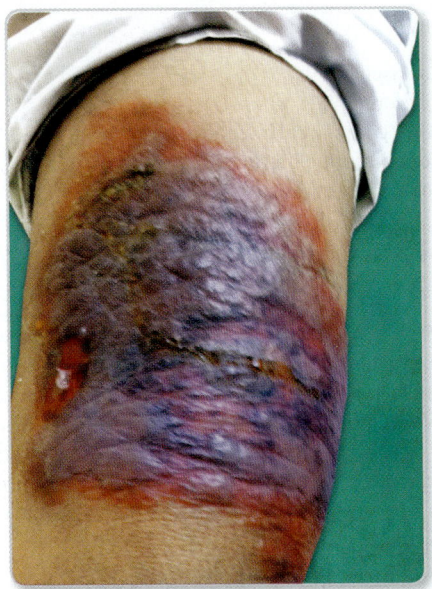

Figure 2.16A: Cellulitis complicated with early changes of necrotizing fasciitis

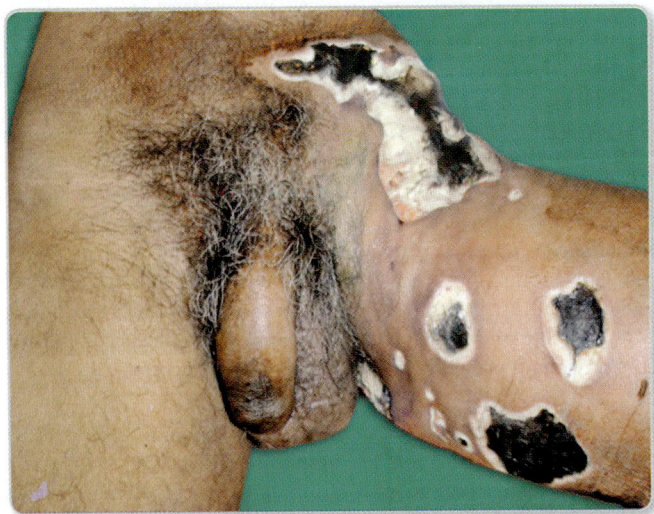

Figure 2.16B: Advanced stage of necrotizing fasciitis in an elderly patient with uncontrolled diabetes mellitus

Clinical Clues

- Woody hard consistency extending beyond the area of apparent involvement is characteristic (unlike the yielding nature of the subcutaneous tissue in cellulitis and erysipelas).
- In presence of an open wound, probing with a blunt instrument allows easy dissection along the fascial planes far beyond the wound margin.

Other clinical pointers to suspect deeper tissue involvement:

- Systemic toxicity, often with altered sensorium.
- Presence of bullous lesions.
- Evidence of ecchymosis/skin necrosis.
- Failure to respond to initial adequate antibiotic therapy.

Peroperative clues of NF:

- There is discharge of a thin, brownish exudate from the wound.
- Fascia looks dull gray in color with stringy areas of necrosis.
- Pus is not found even after deep dissection.
- Ability to dissect tissue planes easily with gloved fingers or blunt instruments.

Rapid Laboratory Diagnostic Methods

Clinical diagnosis is most important in making decision in patients with NF. In case of diagnostic difficulty, CT scan or magnetic resonance imaging of the affected area may be undertaken, which reveals edema fluid along the fascial plane.

Differential Diagnosis

- Cellulitis and erysipelas
- Purpura fulminans (in early stage)
- Gas gangrene

Management

Patient must be managed in ICU.

Choice of antibiotics in NF is to be decided depending upon the causative organism (**Table 2.5**).

- Appropriate parenteral antibiotics as per culture sensitivity report of the pus from the primary lesion.
- If initial culture sensitivity report is not available, material is obtained from deeper tissue and sent to laboratory. Antibiotics are changed accordingly.
- Surgical debridement is to be undertaken as early as possible; it need to be repeated several times at the interval of 2 to 3 days, till there is no more necrotic tissue.

Meningococcemia

Introduction

Meningococcemia or acute meningococcal septicemia is a fulminating illness caused by infection due to *Neisseria meningitidis*. Outbreaks of meningococcal disease may occur in closed communities and nasopharyngeal carriage is common in this situation. Though it is not primarily a dermatological illness, the characteristic skin lesions may occur in 40 to 90% cases and identification of skin lesions at the early stage of the disease may be life saving.

Why the Disease is an Emergency?

- Meningococcemia may be associated with meningitis (58%) and/or encephalitis.
- AIPF (due to acquired protein C deficiency) and DIC may follow (mortality rate > 50%). There is a strong correlation between extent of protein C deficiency and the negative clinical outcome.
- Myocardial dysfunction and acute adrenal hemorrhage (Waterhouse-Friderichsen syndrome) are the other fatal complications.

Table 2.5: Choice of antibiotics in necrotizing fasciitis

Type	Organism	Usual regimen	Alternative regimen
Monomicrobial infection	S. pyogenes	Penicillin (2–4 MU, 4–6 hourly, IV) + clindamycin (600–900 mg/kg, 8 hourly, IV)	
	S. aureus	Nafcillin/oxacillin (1–2 mg, every 4 hourly, IV) OR Cefazolin (1 g, 2 hourly, IV) OR Clindamycin (600–900 mg/kg, 8 hourly, IV)	MRSA- Vancomycin (30 mg/kg/day, 2 divided doses, IV)
	Clostridium sp	Clindamycin (600–900 mg/kg, 8 hourly, IV) OR Penicillin (2–4 MU, 4–6 hourly, IV)	

Contd...

Contd...

Type	Organism	Usual regimen	Alternative regimen
Polymicrobial infection	S. pyogenes, S. aureus, Gram negative coliform bacteria, Anaerobes	Ampicillin + sulbactam (1.5–3g, 6–8 hourly, IV) OR Piperacillin + tazobactam (3.37g, 6–8 hourly, IV) + clindamycin (600–900 mg/kg, 8 hourly, IV) + ciprofloxacin (400 mg, 12 hourly, IV) OR Imipenem + cilastatin (1 g every 6–8 hourly, IV OR Meropenem (1 g 8 hourly, IV) OR Ertapenem (1 g/day)	cefotaxime (2 g, 6 hourly, IV) + Metronidazole (500 mg, 6 hourly, IV) OR clindamycin (600–900 mg/kg, 8 hourly, IV)

Population at Risk

Children < 10 years of age are the common sufferers. Adults may be affected rarely, especially during epidemic. Children or adults with complement deficiency either inherited or acquired (SLE) are at higher risk of meningococcemia.

Poor prognostic factors on admission are as follows:
- Hypothermia
- Hypotension and shock
- Acidosis
- Purpura fulminans
- Presence of petechiae for < 12 hours, hyperpyrexia and absence of meningitis at admission are indicators of rapid progression.

Clinical Presentation

The child is febrile, associated with malaise, headache and joint pain. There may be features of meningismus and altered sensorium. Early skin lesions are transient, faint, maculopapular rash involving trunk, extremities, palms and soles (**Figure 2.17A**). Subsequently these lesions become petechial with irregular border and smudged appearance **(Figure 2.17B).** Sometimes the lesions are extensive, larger, hemorrhagic, with central necrosis (suggillations) and vesiculation. In presence of purpura fulminans, large, grayish black geographic areas of necrosis appear over pressure points (**Figure 2.17C**).

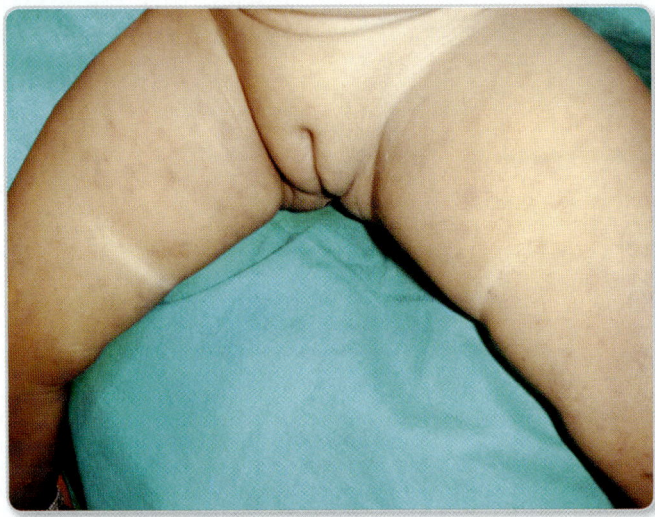

Figure 2.17A: Faint, erythematous, macular rash of meningococcemia

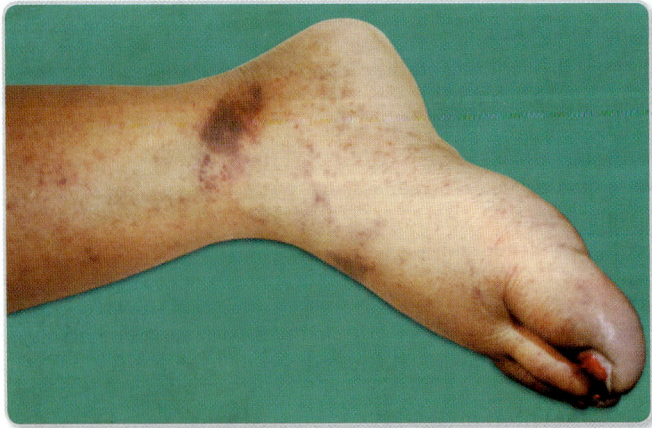

Figure 2.17B: Petechial rash of meningococcemia with irregular border and coalescence

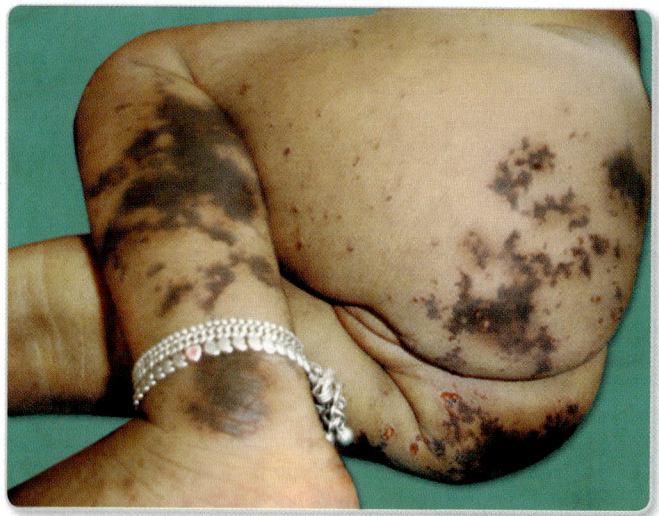

Figure 2.17C: Purpura fulminans in a case of meningococcal meningitis

Clinical Clues

Generalized petechial rash (with irregular border and central dusky area of necrosis) in a febrile child with altered sensorium should raise the suspicion of meningococcemia. Identifying typical skin lesions is one way of early diagnosis of meningococcemia.

Rapid Laboratory Diagnostic Methods

Supportive tests:
- Total and differential leukocyte count (polymorphonuclear leukocytosis with band forms).
- Platelet count (thrombocytopenia in presence of DIC).
- Raised ESR.
- Urinalysis (proteinuria/hematuria).
- Raised CRP.
- Coagulation profile if DIC is suspected.

Confirmatory tests:
- Blood culture (positive almost in 100% cases of acute meningococcemia).
- Cerebrospinal fluid analysis (in presence of meningismus).
- Gram stain of aspirate from skin lesions (positive in 50–80% cases)/CSF.
- Detection of capsular polysaccharide by rapid latex agglutination in CSF in suspected cases (especially if culture is negative as in partially treated cases).

Differential Diagnosis

- Viral exanthematous illness.
- Rocky mountain spotted fever.
- Drug-induced maculopapular rash.
- Subacute bacterial endocarditis.
- Acute rheumatic fever.
- Systemic vasculitis.

Management

These children must be managed in ICU by a well coordinated team of physicians from various specialties.

Appropriate antibiotic therapy;

- Intravenous injection of penicillin G (4 million units × 4 hourly × 7 days).
- In areas where penicillin resistant meningococci is prevalent, intravenous injection of 3rd generation cephalosporins (ceftriaxone, 100 mg/kg/24 hours OR cefotaxime, 200 mg/kg/24 hours) for 7 days.
- In adult patients with penicillin allergy, injection chloramphenicol 1g IV, 6 hourly, may be administered.
- Aggressive management of shock with fluid replacement, along with repeated infusion of colloids (40 ml/kg). Inotropic drugs must be added to ensure perfusion to all vital organs. If patients respond poorly to inotropic agents and there is persistent hypotension, adrenal insufficiency should be suspected and supplementation with hydrocortisone must be done.
- Maintenance of electrolyte and acid-base balance.
- Management of purpura fulminans.

Requirement of protein C infusion is decided by:

- circulating protein C level,
- severity of coagulopathy,
- clinical features; appearance of new purpuric lesions, which coalesce to form necrotic areas, impending peripheral gangrene.

However, protein C replacement therapy is not helpful unless the general resuscitation and management of infection is optimum.

It must also be supplemented by anticoagulant therapy, heparinization followed by warfarin. Usually the coagulopathy is reversed by 5 days, evidenced by increase in platelet count, fibrinogen level and decreased circulating D-dimer level.

- Debridement of necrosed skin and gangrenous areas.

Disseminated Gonococcal Infection

Introduction

The other name for disseminated gonococcal infection (DGI) is 'acute dermatitis arthritis syndrome'. It is a systemic complication of acute gonorrhea due to bacteremia occurring among 0.5–3% of untreated cases, but incidence may be higher in endemic areas. Genitourinary symptoms may be minimal or absent, and hence DGI may be misdiagnosed initially or remain undiagnosed in many cases. In presence of visceral involvement, it is termed as 'complicated DGI.' DGI is typically caused by AHU-auxotypes of *N.gonorrhoeae*.

Why the Disease is an Emergency?
- Patient presents with acute polyarthritis.
- Gonococcal bacteremia may result in following complications:
  - Perihepatitis (Fitz-Hugh Curtis syndrome) and hepatitis.
  - Endocarditis (1–3%); extensive valve damage mostly involving the aortic valve, resulting in progressive aortic incompetence and heart failure. This complication was commoner in the pre-antibiotic era.
  - Acute gonococcal meningitis; other clinical features of disseminated gonococcal infection may be absent.
  - Epidural abscess (rare).

Population at Risk
- Women are more at risk to develop disseminated gonococcal infection and in 50% cases the clinical features start 7 days post-menstruation.
- Pregnancy may be a risk factor.
- Pharyngeal gonorrhea may be a risk factor.
- Patients with terminal complement component deficiency; inherited or acquired (SLE).

Clinical Presentation
Though there is bacteremia, unlike in case of other pyogenic bacteria, the patient is not clinically toxic. Fever and chill may occur but 40% patients remain afebrile. The classic skin lesions are tender papule or pustules on erythematous base or petechial lesions, distributed sparsely (< 30 in number) over pressure points and distal extremities (finger tips). Sometimes lesions are painless and go unrecognized. In the initial stage, there is arthralgia and synovitis and later polyarthritis typically involving wrists, ankles, knees and metacarpophalangeal joints, but other joints may also be involved. Primary focus of infection may be identified in 70 to 80% patients with disseminated gonococcal infection.

Clinical Clues
In a patient with gonorrhea, appearance of characteristic skin lesions distributed over acral areas along with arthritis involving multiple joints should alert the clinician of the possibility of disseminated gonococcal infection.

Rapid Laboratory Diagnostic Methods
- Blood culture.
- Culture from skin lesions, synovial fluid.
- Culture from primary mucosal infection site, e.g. urethra, cervix or pharynx.

Depending upon culture positivity, patients may be categorized as follows:
   - Proven DGI (50%): Positive culture from otherwise sterile specimen; blood, skin lesions and synovial fluid.
   - Probable DGI (> 80%): Positive culture from genitourinary/pharyngeal mucosa/from sex partner, but negative from sterile specimen.
   - Possible DGI: Negative culture from all sites but appropriate clinical features and therapeutic response.
- Synovial fluid leukocyte count (>25,000/mm^3, suggestive of purulent synovial fluid, >40,000/mm^3, often culture positive, <20,000/mm^3, often culture negative).
- HIV status of the patient must be determined.

Differential Diagnosis
- Reactive arthritis
- Acute rheumatoid arthritis.

Management
- Hospitalization
- Antibiotic therapy: Injection ceftriaxone 1 g IV/24 hours, to be continued till 24 to 48 hours after clinical improvement starts.
  Alternative antibiotics are injection cefotaxime 1g IV 8 hourly
  OR
  Injection ceftizoxime 1 g IV 8 hourly, till 24 to 48 hours after clinical improvement starts.
  Thereafter oral antibiotics should be continued (tablet cefixime 400 mg twice daily) to complete a total therapy for 7 days.
- In presence of meningitis injection ceftriaxone 1 to 2 g administered every 12 hourly for 10 to 14 days.
- In presence of endocarditis, injection ceftriaxone 1 to 2 g administered every 12 hourly for 4 weeks. (In presence of such complications, consultation with infectious disease specialist is desirable).
- All cases of DGI must be treated presumptively for chlamydial infection (cap doxycycline 100 mg twice daily for 2 weeks).
- Sex partner must be identified and treated.

Rickettsial Spotted Fever
Introduction
Rickettsial spotted fever (RSF) is a multisystem infection caused by *Rickettsia rickettsii*, associated with a very high fatality. It is a vector borne (tick) disease and dogs may be the carrier of the tick.

Why the Disease is an Emergency?

There is involvement of lungs (noncardiogenic pulmonary edema), heart (myocarditis, arrhythmia), liver (hepatitis), kidney (renal failure) and CNS (meningismus, altered mental status, seizure, focal deficits, coma). Purpura fulminans and DIC may complicate the course of the disease. Death may ensue due to irreversible shock during dissemination of the organism in CNS and other viscera.

Patients with G6PD deficiency may develop fulminant RSF, in which there is profound coagulopathy and widespread visceral thrombosis leading to death in < 5 days.

Population at Risk

People living in tick-infested geographical areas. Clinical risk factors for fatal outcome include:
- Hepatomegaly and jaundice.
- Stupor.
- Acute renal failure.
- Respiratory distress.
- DIC.

Clinical Presentation

There is an eschar at the site of initial bite of tick. It is a symptom complex comprised of the triad of 'fever, headache and myalgia.' However, at presentation all the three features are observed in only 3% of patients. The characteristic discrete, rose-red, blanchable maculopapular rash (**Figures 2.18A to C**) appears after 3 days of fever and initially involves the wrists

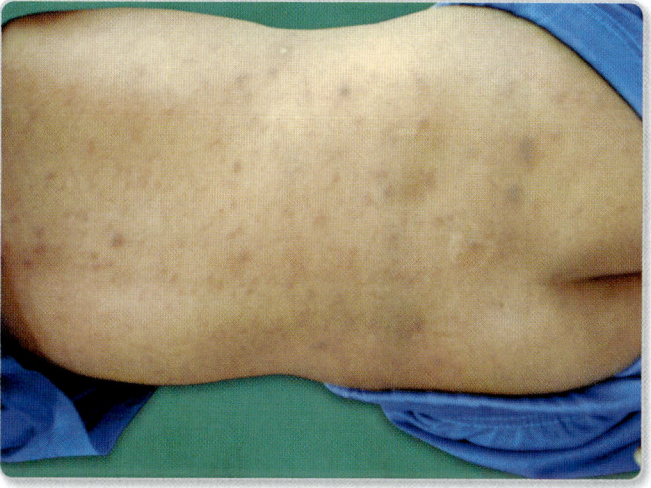

Figure 2.18A: Characteristic rose-red maculopapular rash of rickettsial spotted fever, few lesions attaining petechial character

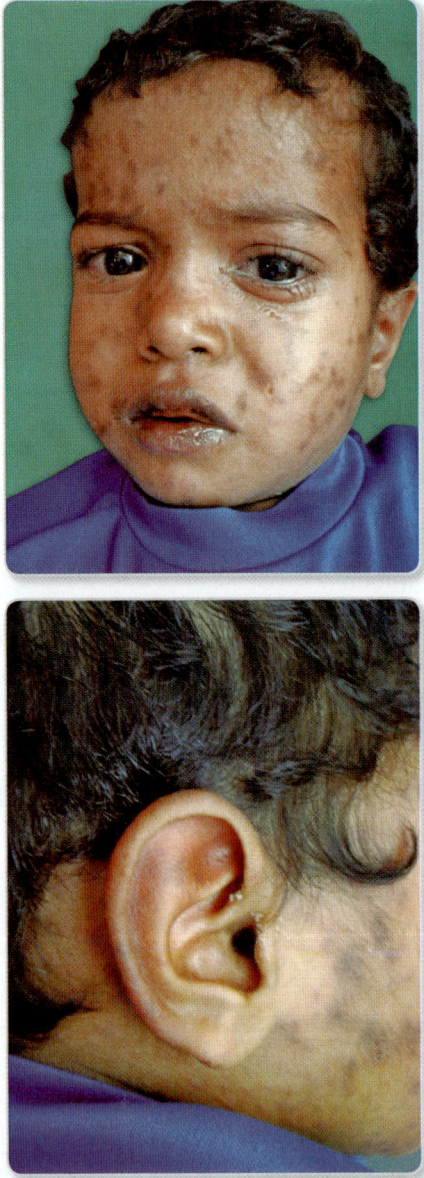

Figures 2.18B and C: Petechial rash of rickettsial spotted fever over face and pinna

and ankles, spreading to palms and soles and thereafter centripetally to involve proximal extremities, trunk and face. The rash is turned petechial by 3 to 4 days, or may coalesce to become ecchymotic. The skin lesions fade slowly over 2 to 3 weeks, sometimes leaving hyperpigmentation. Some patients may not develop the skin rash (spotless RSF, 10–15%). There may be peripheral gangrene involving digits, tip of the nose, ear lobule and genitalia. Hepatosplenomegaly is present in 1/3rd of the patients.

Clinical Clues

In an endemic area of tick infestation, if a patient presents with the classical clinical triad followed by appearance of maculopapular rash (hallmark feature), which turns purpuric, RSF must be suspected. Lesion over palms and soles is a differentiating feature from other exanthematous illnesses.

Rapid Laboratory Diagnostic Methods

- Normal or slightly decreased leukocyte count with a shift to the left (50%).
- Thrombocytopenia (50%).
- Low serum sodium (50%).
- Positive Weil-Felix test (lacks both sensitivity and specificity).
- Serology: A fourfold rise in antibody titer by indirect fluorescent antibody (IFA) assay (acute and convalescent sera) confirms the diagnosis but is time consuming.
- Immunofluorescent staining of skin lesion is a highly sensitive (70%) and specific rapid diagnostic method but not available freely and requires expertise for interpretation.

Differential Diagnosis

- Viral hemorrhagic fevers like dengue fever, chikungunya fever, etc.
- Meningococcemia.
- Initial stage of Stevens-Johnson syndrome/toxic epidermal necrolysis.
- Cutaneous small vessel vasculitis.

Management

- Supportive care of the patients with multiorgan failure, preferably in an ICU.
- Local wound care: If still embedded, the tick has to be removed. Using hand gloves, with the help of a blunt, curved forceps, the tick is grasped as close to the skin as possible and a steady upward pressure is exerted for 3 to 5 minutes causing its dislodgement. Jerking/twisting of the forceps may cause breakage and retaining of its mouth parts in the wound.
- Specific therapy: Doxycycline 100 mg BD X 2 weeks, if patient is able to take orally. This therapy can not be administered in children < 9 years. In patients unable to take orally, parenteral doxycycline or tetracycline may be used. Other drugs with doubtful efficacy are quinolones/azithromycin/clarithromycin.

Dengue Hemorrhagic Fever and Dengue Shock Syndrome

Introduction

Dengue is a mosquito-borne acute, febrile viral illness, which may present in three clinical forms; dengue fever, dengue hemorrhagic fever (DHF) and dengue shock syndrome (DSS). DSS may complicate the course of 20 to 30% cases of DHF. According to WHO grading system of dengue fever, DHF is the grade II illness and DSS comes under grade III and grade IV illnesses.

Why the Disease is an Emergency?

In patients with DHF, there is acute onset hemorrhage both from superficial sites and viscera which may lead to acute hemorrhagic shock. DSS is associated with capillary leak syndrome and acute circulatory failure followed by death. Patients with prolonged shock may develop disseminated intravascular coagulation. Mortality rate associated with DSS is 40 to 50%.

Population at Risk

- As compared to adults, infants and children are more at risk to develop DHF and DSS.
- Superadded infection by a second serotype of dengue virus in a patient with dengue fever (simultaneously/sequentially) is an important risk factor for development of DHF.
- Some infants may develop DHF during primary infection only, if the mother is immune to dengue.

Clinical Presentation

DHF and DSS occur as a complication of dengue fever, occurring during the convalescence period (after 3rd day of fever). At this stage patients may develop sudden deterioration with cold clammy extremities, diaphoresis, circumoral and peripheral cyanosis, restlessness and epigastric pain; there may be purpura, ecchymosis and bleeding from multiple sites (gum bleeding, epistaxis, hematemesis and melena) and subsequently patient may develop acute circulatory failure.

Clinical Clues

- Sudden onset spontaneous bleeding from multiple sites (thrombocytopenia) (**Figure 2.19**) and development of pleural effusion/ascites (sign of increased capillary permeability) in a patient with proved or suspected dengue fever is a clue to the diagnosis of DHF. Bleeding from venipuncture sites may be a common initial finding.

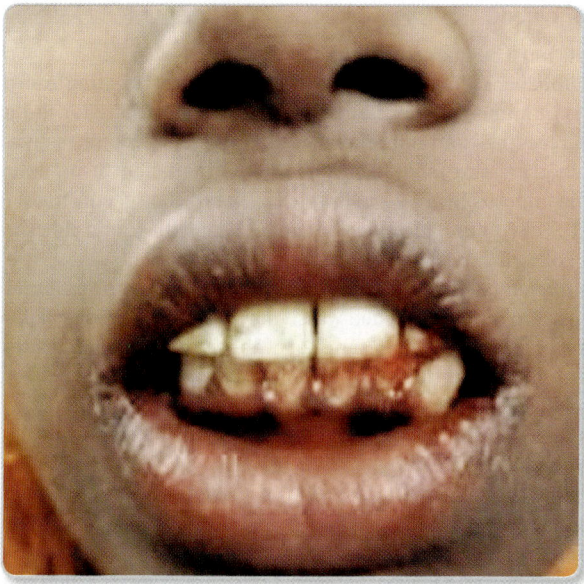

Figure 2.19: Spontaneous gum bleeding in a child with dengue hemorrhagic fever
(*Courtesy:* Dr KA Seetharam, Dermatologist, Guntur)

- If the patient becomes restless with tachycardia, unrecordable blood pressure (hypotension), narrow pulse pressure (≤20 mm Hg) and cold clammy extremities, DSS should be suspected.

Rapid Laboratory Diagnostic Methods
- IgM antibody (detectable after 6–7 days of the onset of illness).
- Pancytopenia with WBC count as low as 2000/mm^3.
- Platelet count (marked thrombocytopenia, < 50,000, in DHF).
- Increased hematocrit (>20% for the age and sex of the patient), suggestive of increased capillary permeability.
- Elevated liver enzymes.
- Prolonged bleeding time, clotting time, prothrombin time, partial thromboplastin time.
- Chest X-ray (pleural effusion).
- Ultrasonography abdomen (ascites).

Differential Diagnosis
- Other viral hemorrhagic fevers.
- Meningococcemia.
- RSF.
- Hematological disorders with acute thrombocytopenia, e.g. acute leukemia, idiopathic thrombocytopenic purpura.

Management

Patients must be managed in an ICU.

Immediate recognition of DHF/DSS in a patient suffering from dengue fever is of immense importance and may be life saving for the patient. Subtle bleedings and minimal alteration of hemodynamic status (pulse rate, blood pressure) should never be ignored as patient resuscitation may become impossible in a very short time. There is no specific treatment for DHF/DSS. Symptomatic management of hemorrhage and shock must be done. Following measures should be undertaken:

- Maintenance of adequate fluid volume and electrolyte levels (overhydration must be avoided which may precipitate cardiac failure).
- Oxygen inhalation in presence of cyanosis or respiratory distress.
- Fresh blood transfusion in presence of significant active bleeding or rapidly decreasing hematocrit.
- Platelet concentrate transfusion in presence of significant thrombocytopenia and bleeding.
- Fresh frozen plasma transfusion in presence of disseminated intravascular coagulation.
- Management of shock.

Following initial recovery, patient must be closely monitored for 48 hours as shock may recur. Early and intensive supportive management may reduce the mortality of DSS to <1%.

BACTERIAL TOXIN MEDIATED ILLNESSES

A. Staphylococcal scalded skin syndrome
B. Toxic shock syndrome
C. Scombroid fish poisoning

Staphylococcal Scalded Skin Syndrome

Introduction

Staphylococcal scalded skin syndrome (SSSS) is a staphylococcal toxin mediated illness (exfoliative toxins, ET-A, ET-B, ET-D) characterized by widespread peeling off of skin. There is an evident or occult focus of infection from where the toxins liberated by the organism are hematogenously spread.

Why the Disease is an Emergency?

Widespread denudation of the skin may lead to fluid and electrolyte imbalance and hypothermia (acute skin failure). These complications may lead to fatality especially in premature infants.

Secondary gram negative infection (*P. aeruginosa*) and septicemia are other complications and these risks are also higher in premature infants.

Population at Risk

SSSS is an illness of childhood. Premature neonates are especially prone to develop SSSS, as they are unable to excrete the exotoxin through kidney, causing perpetuation of the clinical features. Adult patients may also be affected and immunosuppressed states and chronic alcoholism are the predisposing factors.

Clinical Presentation

Usually there is an untreated primary focus of infection, involving pharynx, conjunctiva, anterior nares, skin, perineum or umbilical stump in neonates. Fever, irritability, diffuse erythema, scarlatiniform rash and skin tenderness are the initial clinical features, followed by formation of flaccid bullae which rupture easily to leave painful erosions. In the initial stages, the bullae may be localized to one body part. Subsequently there is widespread involvement and the patient may develop erythroderma **(Figure 2.20A)**. Nikolsky's sign is positive **(Figure 2.20B)**. There is tissue-paper like wrinkling of the skin over face and flexures.

Clinical Clues

Initially, there is an erythema of the skin which gives the child a scalded appearance. In well-established disease, there is separation of the perioral crusts leaving behind radial fissures around the mouth, which is typical of SSSS **(Figure 2.20C)**.

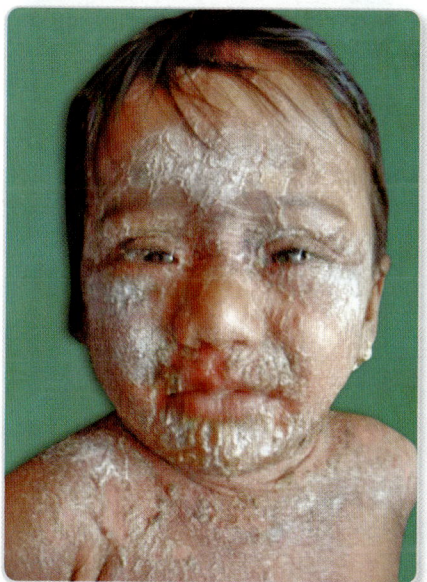

Figure 2.20A: Staphylococcal scalded skin syndrome resulting in erythroderma in a child

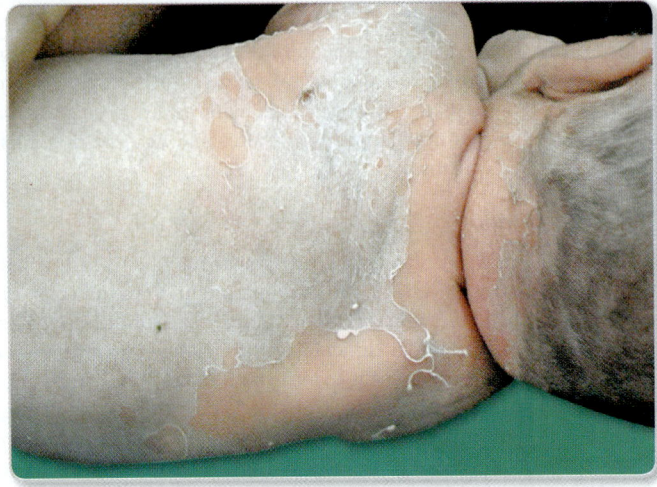

Figure 2.20B: Positive Nikolsky's sign in an infant with staphylococcal scalded skin syndrome

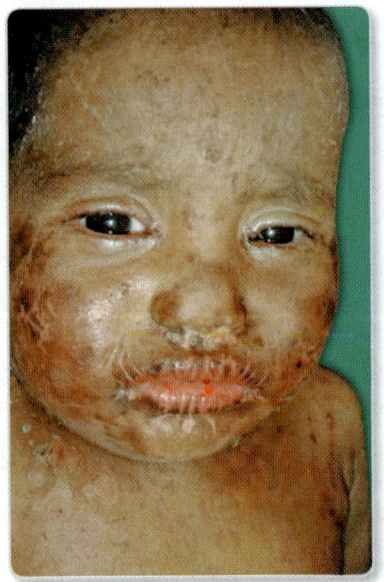

Figure 2.20C: Radial fissures in perioral region in a child with staphylococcal scalded skin syndrome

Rapid Laboratory Diagnostic Methods
- Tzanck preparation from a freshly denuded area reveals many acantholytic cells without inflammatory cells.
- Complete hemogram.
- Blood culture (positive in < 5% of pediatric patients as compared to >50% adults).

Differential Diagnosis
- Bullous impetigo.
- Toxic epidermal necrolysis.
- Hereditary mechanobullous disorders.
- Bullous mastocytosis.

Management
Since SSSS is a toxin mediated illness, there is controversy regarding use of antibiotics in this condition. However, early administration of antibiotic may be helpful in treating the active focus of the infection and may even halt the progression of the disease.
- Parenteral antistaphylococcal antibiotic (cloxacillin, flucloxacillin) for 7 to 10 days.
- Alternative drugs are clindamycin and cefotaxime.
- If there is secondary gram negative infection, injection gentamicin/amikacin may be added.
- In presence of acute skin failure, the child must be admitted in DICU and managed accordingly.

Toxic Shock Syndrome
Introduction
Toxic shock syndrome (TSS) is a staphylococcal or streptococcal exotoxin (superantigen) mediated multisystemic illness. Two variants, menstrual and nonmenstrual TSS has been described. Menstrual TSS has been associated with tampon use (staphylococcal) and is a rarity now a day. TSS occurring in recent times is mostly of nonmenstrual origin.

Mortality associated with nonmenstrual TSS is far lower (2%–5%) as compared to menstrual TSS (13–15%), frequent in the past. However, at present the estimated risk of fatality of nonmenstrual TSS is two times higher than that of menstrual TSS because of under diagnosis of the former condition. Streptococcal TSS (STSS) is not menstruation associated and the primary focus is invasive soft tissue infection.

Why the Disease is an Emergency?
TSS may cause fatal complications like:
- Septicemia, hypotension and altered sensorium.
- ARDS.

- Thrombocytopenia and DIC.
- Acute renal failure and other organ failure.

Population at Risk

Staphylococcal TSS: Tampon-associated menstrual cases (rarity now), were rampant among women of child-bearing age. At present, staphylococcal TSS may occur irrespective of age and sex, but with underlying conditions;
- Postsurgical.
- AIDS.
- Upper respiratory tract infection (influenza) with superadded infection by *S. aureus*.

However, there is an overall female preponderance in staphylococcal TSS as menstrual cases continue to occur.

Streptococcal TSS:
- Occur irrespective of age and sex, in patients with invasive soft tissue infection.
- May occur in children with varicella.

Clinical Presentation

There is an initial infective focus followed by fever, diffuse, erythematous skin rash, mucosal hyperemia (oral, vaginal, conjunctival) and hypotension. In well-established cases, evidence of systemic involvement is prominent, e.g. vomiting and/or diarrhea, myalgia, arthralgia, altered sensorium and adult respiratory distress syndrome. Peeling of palms and soles may occur 1 to 2 weeks after the onset of the illness.

Clinical Clues

The diffuse, non-pruritic, blanchable erythema of skin with the characteristic rough texture (sand paper-like) is the hallmark feature of TSS and constitutes one of the major diagnostic criteria. Associated mucosal hyperemia is a pointer to the diagnosis. The skin lesions subside by 10 days with typical desquamation of hands and feet. Streptococcal TSS is associated with very high incidence of bacteremia and hypotension. The clinical pointer to the diagnosis of Streptococcal TSS is invasive soft tissue infection which is almost always present.

Rapid Laboratory Diagnostic Methods

The diagnosis is mostly clinical; however, series of investigations are required to know the extent of organ involvement as well as for patient monitoring and follow-up. Following investigations are required:
- Total and differential leukocyte count, platelet count.
- Arterial blood gas estimation.
- Serum electrolytes (including calcium and phosphorus).

- Renal function test.
- Liver function test.
- Creatinine phosphokinase (CPK) level (in presence of myositis/fasciitis).
- Urinalysis (sterile pyuria and RBC casts).
- Chest X-ray (ARDS).
- Blood culture (60–100% of STSS patients have bacteremia).
- Culture from involved soft tissue (STSS).

Differential Diagnosis

Staphylococcal TSS:
- Scarlet fever,
- SSSS,
- Kawasaki disease,
- Early stage of SJS-TEN,
- RSF,
- Rubeola,
- Meningococcemia,
- Maculopapular drug rash.

Streptococcal TSS: In addition to the above differential diagnosis, STSS may be mistaken for few other conditions associated with soft tissue involvement. These are as follows:
- Thrombophlebitis,
- Venous gangrene,
- Acute occlusive vasculopathy,
- Soft tissue contusion,
- Hematoma.

Management

Patients with TSS must be managed in an ICU.
- Maintenance of airways (endotracheal intubation and mechanical ventilation) and hemodynamic status if the patient is critically ill.
- In presence of hypotension, aggressive fluid replacement is necessary, with administration of vasopressors and inotropic agents.
- Removal of any potential source of the organism (collected pus as in abscess, foreign bodies like vaginal tampon, nasal pack, wound drain, etc).
- Appropriate administration of anti-staphylococcal antibiotics which does not influence the disease course but prevent recurrence of disease. In STSS, aggressive treatment with parenteral anti-streptococcal antibiotic is required. When the pathogen is unknown, choice of antibiotic should be such that these provide coverage for both the organisms. Clindamycin may be added in addition to the standard antibiotic regimen as it inhibits staphylococcal toxin production (including superantigen).

- Fresh frozen plasma in presence of abnormal coagulation profile.
- IVIg may be used in TSS as it may neutralize the action of superantigen.

Scombroid Fish Poisoning

Introduction

Scombroid fishes are those with dark flesh (tuna, mackerel, bonito, sword fish, etc), rich in amino acid histidine. In contaminated canned scombroid fish, there is bacterial degradation of the histidine (by bacterial histidine decarboxylase enzyme) with release of large amount of histamine. Consumption of this contaminated fish (commonly as tuna salad) results in severe cutaneous and systemic features pertaining to histamine.

Why the Disease is an Emergency?

The onset of the illness is dramatic within minutes to hours of consuming the contaminated fish, simulating fish induced type I hypersensitivity reaction (anaphylaxis). The later is a fatal reaction whereas the former is usually self-limiting. Differentiation is also important as the treatment of both the conditions differ.

Population at Risk

People consuming contaminated canned scombroid fish are at risk of developing symptoms and a large outbreak may occur if the food source is at a common eatery like cafeteria/restaurant.

Clinical Presentation

Widespread erythema of skin appears within several minutes to one hour of consumption of the fish preparation, associated with sweating, palpitation, nausea, vomiting, diarrhea, altered taste, headache and dizziness. The condition persists few hours to days and may be self-limiting.

Clinical Clues

The pointer to this diagnosis is the occurrence of an urticaria-like reaction (erythema without wheal) in several persons following consumption of the same canned fish preparation.

Rapid Laboratory Diagnostic Methods

High histamine level is detected in patient's blood as well as in the consumed fish. Later prick test with fish allergen may be done, which is negative.

Differential Diagnosis

- *Fish allergy:* Type I hypersensitivity due to parvalbumin content of fish (e.g. codfish), manifested by wheal, flare and systemic symptoms.

There is no bacterial contamination of the food. Prick test with fish allergen is positive.
- *Bacterial food poisoning due to fish:* Clinical features are mainly gastrointestinal (vomiting and diarrhea). Prior bacterial contamination is present and food prepared of any type of fish may result in this condition. Prick test with fish allergen is negative.

Management

- High dose intravenous antihistamines, which may have to be repeated. Intravenous steroid is ineffective.
- Preventive measures include:
  - Proper handling and storage of the fish as cooking does not destroy these heat-stable bacterial toxins.
  - Immediate tracing of the contaminated food source to prevent the occurrence of a larger outbreak.

REACTIONS IN LEPROSY

A. Severe neuritis with nerve abscess/impending nerve palsy
B. Severe type 2 reaction

Severe Neuritis with Nerve Abscess/Impending Nerve Palsy

Introduction

Patients with borderline spectrum of leprosy may present with severe form of type 1 reaction presented as:
- Acute pain along the distribution of a peripheral nerve with or without impending paralysis.
- Nerve abscess presenting as erythema, edema and swelling of the involved limb.

Why the Disease is an Emergency?

- Acute neuritis may lead to sudden palsy of an important body part, e.g. foot drop, wrist drop, claw hand (partial/complete), lagophthalmos, and functional impairment.
- Acute neuritis is associated with excruciating pain.

Population at Risk

- Patients with borderline leprosy with involvement of peripheral nerve trunk, like ulnar nerve, common peroneal nerve, branches of facial nerve (in patients having large borderline tuberculoid [BT] patch in periocular location), etc.
- Females and elderly patients are more susceptible to develop type 1 reaction and neuritis.

- Women during initial 6 months after child birth are more at risk of developing neuritis.

Clinical Presentation

Usually patient is a known case of borderline leprosy. Otherwise, a previously undiagnosed case of borderline leprosy may present with acute neuritis for the first time. There is excruciating shooting pain along the distribution of a nerve trunk. In presence of a nerve abscess, the involved limb is diffusely swollen, warm and erythematous with dull aching/throbbing pain.

In both the situations the nerve tenderness is so severe that the patient may not allow the clinician to touch the area.

There may be other features of type 1 reaction like, fever, erythema and swelling of the skin lesions. Testing motor function may reveal evidence of early paralysis

Clinical Clues

- Patient is a known case of borderline leprosy.
- On palpation, the nerve is thick like a cord and tender.
- The abscess is palpable as a diffuse fusiform swelling along the course of the nerve.

Rapid Laboratory Diagnostic Methods

Acute neuritis and nerve abscess in a known patient of leprosy is a clinical diagnosis and does not require laboratory investigation. In some patients of BT or pure neuritic leprosy, in whom the disease was undetected so long and acute neuritis or nerve abscess is the presenting feature, diagnostic confusion may arise. In these situations following investigations may be done:

- Plain X-ray of the involved limb demonstrating soft tissue swelling and rarely calcification along the nerve trunk, suggestive of already damaged nerve.
- Ultrasonography of the involved part shows hypoechoeic areas (swollen, edematous peripheral nerve trunk) with internal soft echo (nerve abscess).

Differential Diagnosis

- Other causes of peripheral neuropathy, causing thickened, tender nerve.
- Acute inflammatory conditions involving extremities/face, e.g. cellulitis.
- Bell's palsy (in cases with lagophthalmos).

Management

In all cases of acute neuritis and nerve abscess, hospitalization of the patient is mandatory. Following measures are taken:

- Bed rest.
- Splinting/collar and cuff sling of the involved upper limb.
- Oral or parenteral analgesic, e.g. diclofenac sodium 50 mg stat and then twice daily till acute pain subsides.
- Injection dexamethasone 2 cc intravenous/intramuscular stat dose and then once daily, till acute pain subsides. Thereafter, it should be substituted with oral prednisolone (40 mg/day, single morning dose) and tapered gradually as per WHO protocol for treatment of type 1 reaction.
- If the patient is on MDT, it should be continued, or started if it is a new case.
- In case of paralysis, active and passive exercise should be started when the acute stage is over.
- Patients with nerve abscess usually respond to conservative therapy as stated above.
- If nerve abscess does not respond to conventional therapy or nerve pain and tenderness continues with worsening of function of a limb, surgical exploration and decompression of the affected nerve should be performed by a surgeon. The affected nerve is exposed and at the point of maximum thickness, multiple longitudinal incisions are made up to the level of epineurium to relieve the pressure upon nerve bundles resulting from inflammatory edema.
- Systemic steroid must be continued during the procedure and thereafter, to prevent postoperative edema.

Severe Type 2 Reaction in Leprosy
Introduction
Patients with lepromatous leprosy (BL/LL) may present with severe form of type 2 reaction. It is an immune complex mediated (type III hypersensitivity) phenomenon causing cutaneous as well as systemic involvement. Occasionally type 2 reaction may be the presenting feature of lepromatous leprosy. Because of varied clinical manifestations, patients with severe type 2 reactions may present to specialists other than dermatologists and result in diagnostic dilemma.

Why the Disease is an Emergency?
Type 2 reaction may be associated with organ-threatening or life-threatening complications as follows:
- Necrotic and ulcerative skin lesions causing damage to deeper tissue.
- Severe arthralgia, restricting patient movement.
- Acute osteitis and myositis, causing incapacitating bone and muscle pain.
- Acute iridocyclitis leading to sudden blindness.
- Acute epididymo-orchitis, resulting in excruciating testicular pain.

- Acute glomerulonephritis.
- Laryngeal (epiglottis/vocal cords) edema causing asphyxia.

Population at Risk
- Patients with BL/LL leprosy with intercurrent infection.
- Women with BL/LL leprosy during pregnancy and postpartum.
- BL/LL patients with sudden psychological stress.

Clinical Presentation
Severe type 2 reaction is an acute, febrile illness associated with severe malaise and crops of extensive erythematous, warm and tender skin lesions, erythema nodosum leprosum (ENL). The skin lesions may be ulcero-necrotic. There may be associated severe bone pain, myalgia and acute-onset testicular pain. These patients may have red eyes with watering, photophobia and sudden diminution of vision. Patients may present with hematuria. In the pre-MDT era, epiglottic edema and asphyxia was common but rare now a day.

Clinical Clues
In presence of classical ENL diagnosis is not difficult for an experienced dermatologist. However, if the patient presents to other departments with multisystemic involvement, diagnosis may be difficult initially. In such situation co-existing deformities of lepromatous leprosy should help to consider the diagnosis of type 2 reaction.

Rapid Laboratory Diagnostic Methods
There is no diagnostic test for type 2 reaction. During acute stage, following laboratory abnormalities may be observed:
- Leukocytosis.
- Raised ESR.
- Elevated CRP.
- Proteinuria and hematuria.
- In presence of acute bone pain, X-ray of the involved bone (usually tibia) helps to differentiate it from acute osteomyelitis.
- In presence of acute testicular pain, ultrasonography of the scrotum and testis helps to differentiate it from other acute conditions like torsion.
- Skin biopsy and histopathological examination (H& E stain and Fite Faracco stain) helps to differentiate ENL from other similar appearing lesions.

Differential Diagnosis
Following conditions must be ruled out during acute stage of the illness:
- Other acute febrile illnesses.
- Acute osteomyelitis (in presence of bone pain).

Dermatological Emergencies

- Torsion of testis (in presence of epididymo-orchitis).
- Erythema nodosum (few lesions of ENL).

Management

All patients with severe type 2 reaction must be hospitalized. Management includes:

- Bed rest.
- If the patient is prostrated, resuscitation should be done using intravenous fluid.
- Specific therapy includes intravenous systemic steroid (injection dexamethasone 2 cc IV stat and thereafter once or twice daily), till the patient is symptomatically well. Once the patient is stable, oral prednisolone (40 mg/day, single morning dose) is to be started and tapered gradually as per WHO protocol for treatment of type 2 reaction. Thalidomide (up to 400 mg/day) should be started along with prednisolone and continued for 3 to 6 months to prevent recurrence.
- NSAIDs (injectable and thereafter oral), if the patient complains of acute pain.
- In presence of underlying focus of infection (e.g. urinary tract infection, upper/lower respiratory tract infection, pyoderma), appropriate antibiotic therapy must be started.
- Anxiolytic and sedative medication during acute stage.
- If the patient is on MDT, it must be continued or started in a newly diagnosed case.
- Supportive management:
    - Acute bone pain: splinting of the limb.
    - Acute neuritis: splinting of the limb.
    - Acute orchitis: scrotal support.
    - Acute iridocyclitis: immediate ophthalmological consultation.
    - Stridor (suggestive of laryngeal edema): tracheostomy.

BITES/STINGS/VENOM

A. Bite by insects of *Hymenoptera* species (bees, wasps, fire ants)
B. Spider (Black widow spider, Brown recluse spider) envenomation
C. Tick paralysis
D. Jellyfish, sea anemones and coral stings

Bite by Insects of *Hymenoptera* Species (Bees, Wasps, Fire Ants)

Introduction

Insects of *Hymenoptera* species possess a sting. Effect of bite by these insects may be variable from mild local reaction to severe anaphylaxis.

Why the Disease is an Emergency?

Bite by insects of *Hymenoptera* species may produce IgE mediated immediate type of hypersensitivity reaction (anaphylaxis). Hence, the cumulative effect of multiple bites by these insects may be fatal, especially in children.

Population at Risk

Professional bee handlers.

Clinical Presentation

The reaction to bite or stings of these insects may be local or generalized. Local reaction is due to injection of pharmacologically active substances and manifests as intense pain, erythema and inflammatory edema, which may subside in few hours. The widespread systemic features (anaphylaxis) consist initially of intense pruritus, urticaria and angioedema; thereafter, patient may develop flushing, headache, vomiting and diarrhea, stridor, palpitation, hypotension and shock. The systemic features may be of varying severity, which is intensified after repeated bites.

Clinical Clues

History of seeing the insect while inflicting bite injury is often available, and helps in diagnosis. Sometimes close inspection of the site of bite may give a clue to the causative insect; fire ant bite usually occurs as clustered papules each of which may be marked by 2 minute hemorrhagic puncta. The fully developed lesions are umbilicated pustules on erythematous and edematous base.

Differential Diagnosis

Drug/food induced anaphylaxis.
Acute urticaria/angioedema.

Management

Mild local reaction is treated with oral antihistamine. Management protocol for anaphylaxis has been described earlier.

Spider Bite (Arachnidism)

Introduction

Among various species of spiders, only few can inflict fatal bite to human beings. The two most dreadful types are 'black widow spider' and 'brown recluse spider.' 'Arachnidism' refers to the symptomatology arising from spider bite.

Black widow spider (Latrodectus mactans) bite (Latrodectism):

Why the Disease is an Emergency?
The venom of *Latrodectus sp* is considered as one of the most potent toxins. The symptoms may persist for several days and unless treated, it is fatal in children and elderly.

Population at Risk
People using outdoor lavatories (in the past), as it is a common habitat of the spider.

Clinical Presentation
The female spider bites only in self-defence. Initial bite is painless but progressive, generalized pain is experienced thereafter along with systemic features like severe abdominal colic, profuse sweating, lethargy, paraesthesia, incoordination and paralysis.

Clinical Clues
Identification of the spider, if noticed, confirms the diagnosis. The female spider has a shiny black body with leg span of about 5 cm. The site of the bite is erythematous and edematous topped with puncta.

Differential Diagnosis
- Other spider/insect bites.

Management
- Management of symptoms.
- Species specific antivenom.

Brown recluse spider (Loxosceles reclusa) bite (Loxoscelism):

Introduction
Loxoscelism is the symptom complex arising from brown recluse spider bite. These spiders are present in all geographic locations. Females, the usual biters are larger in size and more venomous than the male spiders. Brown recluse spider has a nocturnal biting habit, mostly in summer season. Majority of the bites are uneventful but it may be severe in 10% cases, some of which may be fatal. Two clinical variants of loxoscelism are known:
- Cutaneous loxoscelism, the commoner form with mild clinical features.
- Viscerocutaneous loxoscelism, which may lead to fatality.

Why the Disease is an Emergency?
The viscerocutaneous variant of the disease is associated with massive intravascular hemolysis resulting in hematuria, hemoglobinuria, jaundice,

rhabdomyolysis, and severe constitutional symptoms. Thrombocytopenia is the commonest cause of death. Rarely DIC may occur.

Clinical Presentation

Cutaneous loxoscelism: The common presentation is the localized necrotic cutaneous lesion. The bite is usually painless but shortly there is intense pain with wide area of erythema and edema (**Figures 2.21A to C**); the biting site is identified as a tricolor target lesion (central blue/purple

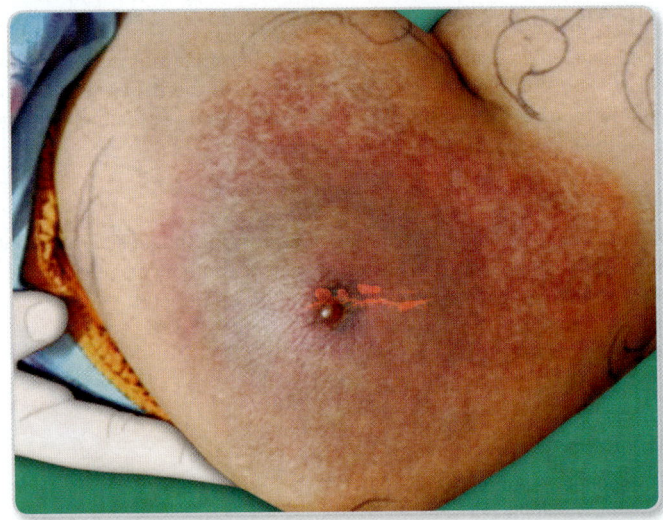

Figure 2.21A: Cutaneous loxoscelism (tricolor target lesion)

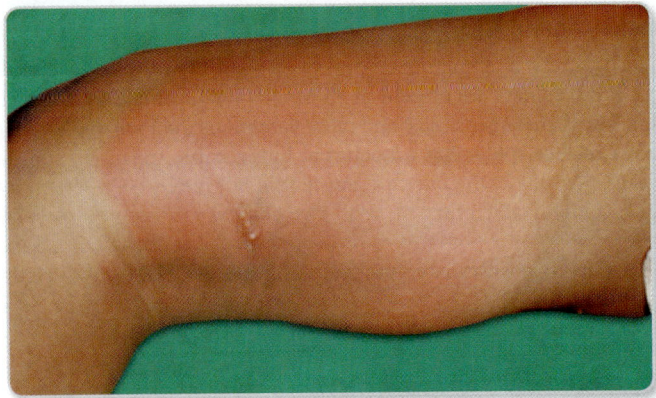

Figure 2.21B: Diffuse erythema in cutaneous loxoscelism; vesicles indicate the site of bite

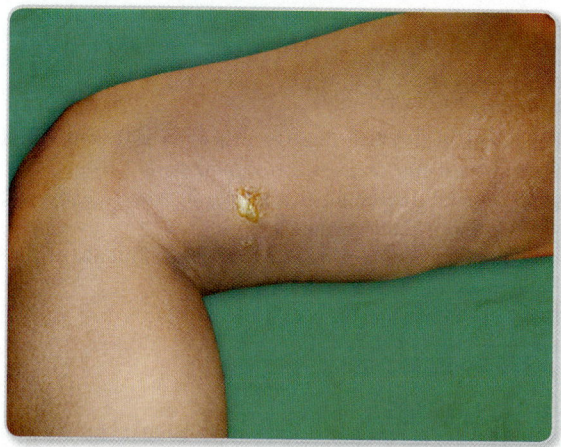

Figure 2.21C: Cutaneous loxoscelism; 10 days following treatment with dapsone (The patient in Figure 2.21B)

necrotic area, surrounded by white ischemic zone and the erythematous zone). Thereafter, there is an eschar formation at the center and the healing time is very prolonged. Mild systemic features may be present.

Viscerocutaneous loxoscelism: Within 2 to 4 days of bite, the patient develops fever, chill, malaise, myalgia, maculopapular rash, nausea and vomiting. The course may be complicated by intravascular hemolysis, acute renal failure and DIC.

Clinical Clues

Identification of the spider, if noticed, confirms the diagnosis. Its body is tan/brown in color with a dark brown violin-like mark on the dorsal aspect of the cephalothorax (fiddle-back/violin spider). The typical targetoid 'red-white-blue' sign at the site of biting followed by eschar formation is characteristic.

Rapid Laboratory Diagnostic Methods

- Complete hemogram with platelet count.
- Urinalysis.
- In presence of DIC, following tests should be done:
    - Prothrombin time,
    - Partial thromboplastin time,
    - Fibrinogen and fibrin degradation product.

Differential Diagnosis

- Other arthropod bite.
- Cellulitis.

- Cutaneous anthrax.
- Fixed drug eruption.

Management

Viscerocutaneous loxoscelism must be treated in ICU with symptomatic management of systemic features. Renal failure and DIC must be treated accordingly. Specific antivenom is available in some countries, but not much is known about its effectiveness.

Course of cutaneous loxoscelism may be self-limiting. In acute stage it may be treated with,

- *R*ICE therapy, consisting of:
  - *R*est
  - *I*ce Compress
  - *E*levation of the part
- Dapsone/colchicine may be helpful in reducing progressive necrosis.
- Antihistamine, NSAIDS, tetanus prophylaxis, antibiotics.
- Surgical debridement if there is a large necrotic area.

Tick Paralysis

Introduction

Feeding tick of certain species may result in this illness. The offending species differs in various regions. Neurotoxin released by the tick, which acts at the neuromuscular junction is responsible for development of paralysis.

Why the Disease is an Emergency?

Occasionally, it may progress to bulbar palsy, respiratory failure and death.

Population at Risk

Children are more commonly affected.

Clinical Presentation

Ascending flaccid paralysis is the usual presenting feature (**Figure 2.22**).

Clinical Clues

Detection of the feeding tick attached on patient's skin.

Differential Diagnosis

Other neurological disorders causing acute palsy.

Management

Removal of the feeding tick completely reverses the condition.

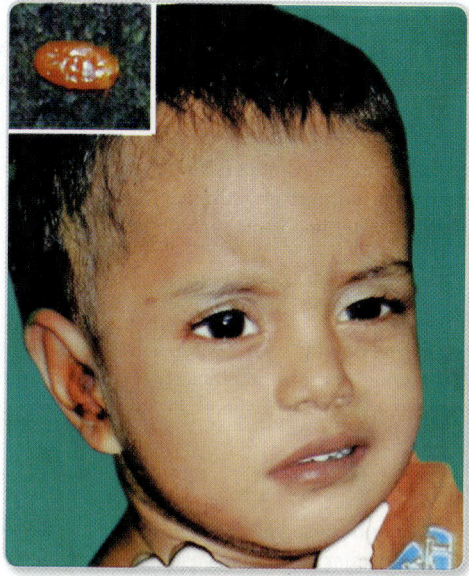

Figure 2.22: Tick paralysis (right sided facial paralysis due to tick bite; inset: the feeding tick removed from right pinna) *(Courtesy: Dr MM Patil, Pediatrician, Bijapur)*

Envenomation by Jellyfish, Sea Anemones and Coral

Introduction

Marine creatures like jellyfish/sea anemones/corals may be important source of serious envenomation for people coming in physical contact with them. Most of these organisms bear tentacles with series of stinging cells (nematocysts) which eject venom when in contact with the human skin. The toxic effect of envenomation by these organisms is variable from local lesions to fatal systemic effects.

Why the Disease is an Emergency?

Envenomation by these organisms causes intense local pain at the site of contact with the nematocysts. Venoms from some species may cause severe systemic effects (hemolysis, acute renal failure) and eventually death.

Population at Risk

- Sea swimmers (amateur or occupational)
- Occupational handlers working in marine aquarium.

Clinical Presentation

Linear beaded wheals at the site of the contact associated with severe pain are the presenting feature. The center of the lesions may become whitish and necrotic or these may become vesiculo-bullous (fire coral). Subsequently there may be partial/full thickness necrosis at the site. With some species, the lesions may be persistent, in the form of recurrent or generalized wheals or chronic granulomatous and lichenoid eruptions (fire coral). Serious systemic effects include hemolysis and acute renal failure.

Clinical Clues

Linear beaded wheals along with severe pain in a sea swimmer are diagnostic. Depending upon the tentacle type, other patterns of initial lesions may be seen, e.g. large wheals in 'cross-hatched' or 'frosted-ladder' pattern.

Differential Diagnosis

- Seabather's eruption caused by the same organisms due to accidental trapping of these under swimming costume and the lesions are more concentrated along the tightly fitted areas.
- Swimmer's itch, caused by cercarial organisms.

Management

- Protective 'stinger suit'
- First aid management with vinegar washes of the local area at the earliest possible (only in cases of cnidarian stings), which prevents discharge of venom from nematocysts.
- Symptomatic management of systemic features, if present.
- Antivenom is available for some species.

■ METABOLIC DISORDERS

A. Neonatal biotin deficiency
B. Acrodermatitis enteropathica

Neonatal Biotin Deficiency

Introduction

It is an autosomal recessive disorder of biotin metabolism, manifesting during the first 3 months of life, resulting from inborn deficiency of the enzyme holocarboxylase synthetase.

Why the Disease is an Emergency?

Metabolic acidosis, ketosis, seizures and coma are the life-threatening situations arising in these babies.

Clinical Presentation

There is acute onset of symptoms, which may be present at birth or appear within the first few weeks of life. Severe, recurrent episodes of vomiting and tachypnea are the presenting features, suggestive of metabolic acidosis. Seizure and coma may lead to death. Skin lesions occur rarely in this variant of the disease and are observed in babies surviving the crisis period of first few days of life. The skin lesions are non-specific, simulating ichthyosis or seborrheic dermatitis.

Clinical Clues

Systemic features are more prominent in these patients and skin lesions are non-specific. However, clinicians should keep this condition as a differential diagnosis in all neonates presenting with features of metabolic acidosis.

Rapid Laboratory Diagnostic Methods

Estimation of urinary organic acid excretion (3-Hydroxyisovaleric acid, 3-HIVA).

Differential Diagnosis

- Organic acidemias (methylmalonic acidemia, propionic acidemia, maple syrup urine disease, glutaric aciduria type I).
- Urea cycle defects (ornithine transcarbamoylase deficiency, citrullinemia, carbamoyl phosphate synthetase deficiency).

Management

Patients must be managed in intensive care unit with close monitoring and symptomatic management for metabolic acidosis and ketosis. Specific therapy includes injection biotin 10 to 40 mg/day.

Acrodermatitis Enteropathica

Introduction

Acrodermatitis enteropathica (AE) is a rare autosomal recessive disorder of zinc metabolism, which manifests during weaning of breast-fed infants. Intestinal zinc absorption is abnormally low in these patients, the specific cause for which is poorly understood. Zinc is an essential component of several metalloenzymes in body and acute zinc deficiency may result in serious metabolic disturbances.

Why the Disease is an Emergency?

In acute stage of AE, the infant is extremely irritable and presents with photophobia, anorexia and voluminous diarrhea. Usually diagnosis is delayed due to absence of any hallmark clinical feature and unless treated promptly, there may be a fatal ending. Infants with acrodermatitis enteropathica are also susceptible to septicemia resulting from secondary infection of skin lesions.

Population at Risk

Onset of the disease occurs during weaning in breast-fed infants (at around 6 months). Non-breastfed infants may develop it earlier. Thereafter, subsequent episodes may occur any time during childhood or in adults if zinc supplementation is not maintained.

Clinical Presentation

Clinical triad of acute stage of AE is diarrhea, periorificial vesicular and crusted dermatitis (**Figures 2.23A to C**) and alopecia. There is associated photophobia and severe anorexia. There may be vesicular lesions on palms and soles. In children with delayed diagnosis, the dermatitis may be disseminated to complicate the clinical picture. The diarrhea is copious, frothy and foul smelling. Almost total alopecia may be present.

Clinical Clues

An irritable infant with periorificial dermatitis, sparse hair and diarrhea should alert the clinician of the diagnosis of AE.

Rapid Laboratory Diagnostic Methods

- Serum zinc level; to be done along with serum albumin level as low serum albumin may falsely indicate a low serum zinc level. Low serum zinc level is confirmatory to the diagnosis of acrodermatitis enteropathica. In certain variant of the disease, (presence of a

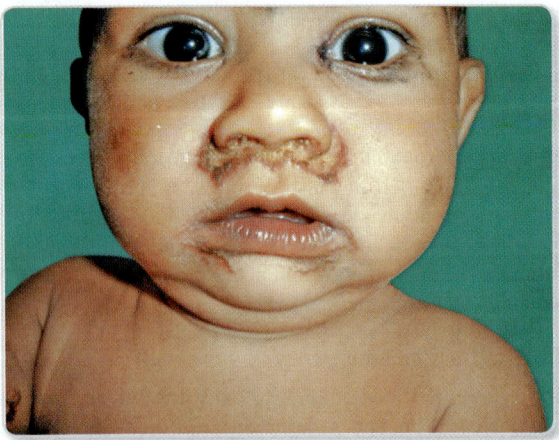

Figure 2.23A: Perioral and perinasal lesions in an infant with acrodermatitis enteropathica

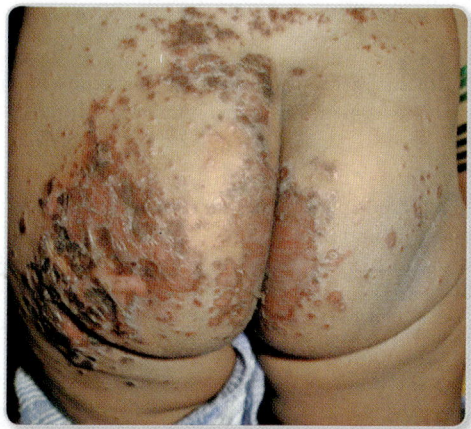

Figure 2.23B: Perianal crusted lesions in an infant with acrodermatitis enteropathica

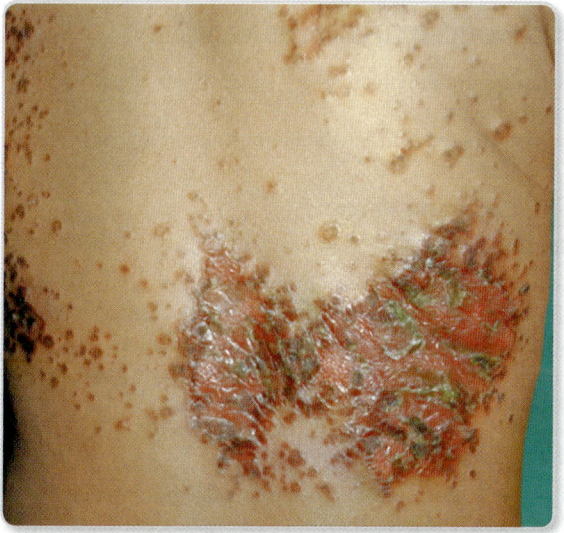

Figure 2.23C: Crusted lesions over back in an infant with acrodermatitis enteropathica

different intestinal zinc-binding ligand, which is unable to release zinc at cellular level) serum zinc level may be normal.
- Serum alkaline phosphatase level may give approximate idea about serum zinc level (if facility for estimation of serum zinc is not available). It remains low in zinc deficient state (reference value 145–420 U/L, for children aged 1–9 years).

Differential Diagnosis
- Impetigo contagiosa.
- Heritable organic acidurias (propionic acidemia, methylmalonic acidemia, maple syrup urine disease, etc.).

Management
- If oral feeding is possible, oral zinc sulfate syrup (2–5 mg/kg/day in 2–3 divided doses) is administered before meals. Total dose should not exceed 50 mg/day in infants and 150–200 mg/day in older children). The first evidence of effective treatment of acute stage is improvement of irritability; this may be an indirect confirmation of the diagnosis of AE in doubtful cases (normal serum zinc level).
- If feeding is not possible or the baby is too sick to take orally, parenteral zinc sulfate (0.2–0.3 mg/kg/day) is administered till the acute stage is over and thereafter oral zinc sulfate supplementation is continued.
- Patients diagnosed as AE must take zinc supplementation at minimum required dose throughout life (1–2 mg/kg/day).

DRUG-INDUCED CUTANEOUS NECROSIS

A. Warfarin/coumarin necrosis
B. Heparin necrosis
C. Tissue necrosis due to catecholamine (dopamine/nor adrenaline)

Warfarin/Coumarin Necrosis
Introduction
Extensive area of skin necrosis may be a complication of therapy with warfarin/other coumarin congeners. Anticoagulation with warfarin in the background of heparin induced thrombocytopenia syndrome (HITS) may also precipitate occurrence of skin necrosis. It is a rare condition with prevalence of 0.01–0.1%.

Why the Disease is an Emergency?
Extensive area of cutaneous necrosis may be associated with high morbidity and a fatal outcome.

Population at Risk
- Patients on oral anticoagulant therapy, following receiving an oral loading dose of warfarin.
- People with heterozygous protein C deficiency, antithrombin and factor VII deficiency are prone to develop this condition.
- Perimenopausal obese women, on warfarin treatment for thromboembolic disorder are more common sufferers.

Clinical Presentation

It starts 1 to 10 days (commonly by 3rd–6th day) following initiation of high dose of warfarin.

Initially there is paraesthesia at the site of impending lesions. Thereafter, patients develop one or more symmetrical, painful, erythematous lesions on fatty areas (breasts, buttocks, abdomen, thighs, calves), which rapidly turn ecchymotic and vesicular. It is followed by large areas of cutaneous and subcutaneous necrosis. There is formation of deep ulcers at the pressure points.

Clinical Clues

Within initial few days of high dose warfarin therapy, sudden appearance of necrotic areas on skin with rapid progression should alert the clinician of this diagnosis. Symmetrical involvement of the fatty body parts with areas of necrosis is the clinical pointer to the diagnosis.

Rapid Laboratory Diagnostic Methods

There is no rapid diagnostic method for this condition. The characteristic feature in histopathology of skin is presence of numerous microthrombi, occluding dermal blood vessels, in absence of vascular inflammation and arterial involvement.

Differential Diagnosis

- Calciphylaxis.
- Heparin-induced skin necrosis.
- Purpura fulminans.
- Cryoglobulinemic vasculitis.
- Disseminated intravascular coagulation.
- Necrotizing fasciitis.

Management

Early recognition may halt the extent of tissue damage. Withdrawal or continuation of warfarin does not appear to alter the course of necrosis.
- Patients are provided with supportive treatment with fresh frozen plasma (to restore protein C and protein S) and injection vitamin K.
- Change anticoagulant to heparin.
- Wound care with dressing and debridement.
- Regular change of posture in presence of pressure ulcer.
- In case of involvement of large areas, skin grafting may be required.

Preventive measure include starting warfarin at a lower dose (1–2 mg/day) and increase the dose daily by 1 to 2 mg/day during the critical period (first 1–10 days), to build up the desired dose. Gradual escalation of dose during the initial 10 days keeps the protein C level stable and thus chance of warfarin necrosis is reduced. Otherwise co-administration of unfractionated heparin for initial 5 days of therapy is recommended (heparin bridge).

Heparin-induced Skin Necrosis

Introduction

It is a rare side effect of unfractionated heparin (more common) and low molecular weight heparin at the injection site. It is an immunologically mediated reaction, and few possible mechanisms have been suggested:

- Intravascular thrombosis due to heparin-induced immune aggregation of platelets, 'heparin-induced thrombocytopenia and thrombosis syndrome (HITT).
- Arthus reaction due to formation of antigen-antibody complex in cutaneous blood vessels.
- Incorrect injection technique.
- Persistence of heparin in subcutaneous fat causing tissue damage.

Why the Disease is an Emergency?

If the condition is not diagnosed early, necrosis may develop over large and distant areas, beyond the original site of heparin injection.

Population at Risk

Middle aged women with thrombotic disorders are at risk of developing this side effect of heparin. Other risk factors are diabetes, and patients receiving high dose of antibiotics.

Clinical Presentation

Areas of skin necrosis may occur at the injection site or at a distant area, 6 to 8 days after starting therapy. It may also occur immediately or after several months. Initially there is erythema, edema and pain at the injection site which gradually turns bullous and thereafter necrotic. A clear cut line of demarcation develops from the surrounding area.

Differential Diagnosis

- Warfarin-induced cutaneous necrosis.
- Necrotizing fasciitis.

Management

- Immediate discontinuation of heparin and switch over to another anticoagulant. Avoidance of other heparin containing compounds and devices (line flushes and coated catheters) is also essential.
- The choice of alternative anticoagulant in acute stage should be direct thrombin inhibitor, argatroban. Warfarin must be used with

extreme care in patients with HITT, as it may induce a transient hypercoagulable state.
- Wound dressing.
- Wound debridement and skin grafting if large area is involved.

Tissue Necrosis due to Vasopressors

Introduction

Use of vasopressor agents during treatment of shock may cause direct tissue necrosis due to extravasation or may induce skin lesions at distant body sites and peripheral gangrene even when administered through central venous line. Cutaneous necrosis has been reported in patients on treatment with dopamine, noradrenaline and vasopressin.

Dopamine is a catecholamine, used as intravenous infusion in the treatment of shock of various etiology. At low infusion rate (< 10 µg/kg/minute), it exerts β-adrenergic effect enhancing peripheral perfusion. At high infusion rate (>10 µg/kg/minute), it exerts α-adrenergic effect, causing peripheral vasoconstriction.

Extravasation of dopamine-mixed intravenous fluid may result in severe local vasoconstriction and ischemic tissue injury.

Why the Disease is an Emergency?

Dopamine, noradrenaline or vasopressin extravasation cause severe tissue necrosis resulting in:
- Partial/complete loss of skin.
- Damage of underlying nerve and tendon causing functional impairment.
- Risk of super-added infection of damaged tissue.
- Severe cosmetic disfigurement.

Population at Risk

Patients being treated with IV vasopressor infusion are at risk. In case of dopamine, the chances are more when there is high infusion rate. However, even with low infusion rate, cumulative high concentration achieved at the site of extravasation may induce tissue necrosis.

Clinical Presentation

Tissue necrosis occurs at the site of extravasation of vasopressors (**Figure 2.24**). In severe cases there is total sloughing off of the skin in affected area with exposure and damage of underlying structures.

There are reports of purpuric lesions and hemorrhagic vesicles with administration of noradrenaline (over finger and toe tips), dopamine and vasopressin (over muscular parts of the extremities) even through central venous line in patients with shock.

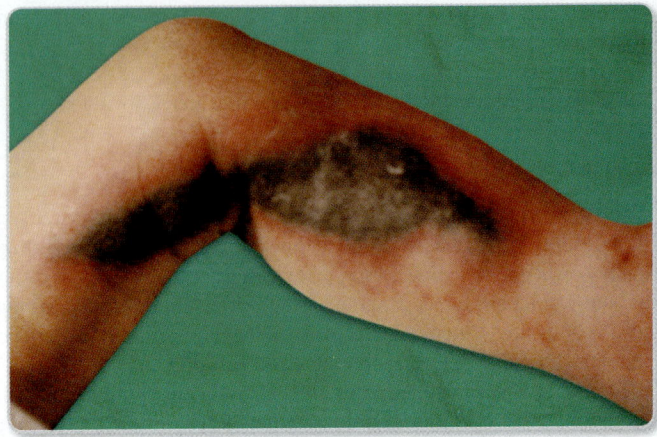

Figure 2.24: Linear tissue necrosis at the site of extravasation of dopamine infusion

Clinical Clues

Appearance of ecchymotic areas which soon become necrotic in patients receiving vasopressor infusion should raise the suspicion of this condition. If the lesion is only at the infusion site, probably it was caused by extravasation. However, occurrence of lesions at other sites should not prevent the clinician from making a diagnosis of vasopressor induced skin necrosis.

Differential Diagnosis

- Purpura fulminans.
- Heparin and warfarin necrosis.
- Early stage of necrotizing fasciitis.

Management

- Immediate withdrawal of the drip containing vasopressor drug if it is still running at the site of extravasation.
- Symptomatic management of the tissue injury with analgesics and prophylactic antibiotic.
- Topical nitroglycerine ointment may be used.
- Local injection of α-adrenenoreceptor blocker phentolamine 5 mg, may be administered.
- Surgical debridement as and when indicated.

Prophylactic Measures

- Vasopressor infusion may be performed through only central venous catheter or through a long IV cannula placed in a large peripheral vein, to avoid extravasation injury.
- A wide bore IV cannula (20 G or more) is recommended for peripheral vasopressor infusion.

- In case of peripheral vasopressor infusion, the infusion site should be inspected frequently to detect early extravasation.

ACUTE GRAFT VERSUS HOST DISEASE

Introduction

Graft versus host disease (GVHD) is a disorder, which arises when immunocompetent T cells from a donor recognize and react against the tissue antigens in an immunocompromised host. It occurs in the following contexts:

- Patients with bone marrow transplantation (BMT) or hemopoietic stem cell transplantation (HSCT).
- Following transfusion of non-irradiated blood/blood components.
- Following peripheral blood stem cell transfer.
- Following materno-fetal transfer of lymphoid cells, particularly in immunodeficient fetus.
- Following solid organ allografting (liver/kidney).

The two types of GVHD are acute and chronic. Incidence of BMT related GVHD is around 50%, which may occur even after autologous BMT (10%).

Why the Disease is an Emergency?

- The skin lesions may be very severe simulating SJS or there may be erythroderma.
- There may be organ involvement like hepatitis and enteritis, and death may occur by 3 weeks time.
- Thrombocytopenia may be present.
- The hyperacute GVHD may present with capillary leak syndrome and shock.
- Mortality in moderate to severe acute GVHD is 50%.

Population at Risk

Patients having BMT/HSCT or blood transfusion.

Clinical Presentation

Acute GVHD usually occurs within 60 days (most often within 4–6 weeks) of BMT. A 'hyperacute' variant may occur within 7–12 days, associated with high mortality. There is fever and a faint, itchy, maculopapular rash starting on face and extremities, which become generalized. Palms and soles are involved and there is desquamation from the involved areas. A nonspecific mucositis is usually present. There is varying morphology of the skin lesions like vesicular/SJS-like/follicular/ulcerative or patient may present with erythroderma. There is associated hepatitis and enteritis giving rise to bloody diarrhea.

Clinical Clues

History of preceding BMT or blood transfusion should lead the clinician to consider acute GVHD as the probable diagnosis.

Rapid Laboratory Diagnostic Methods

- Histopathological examination of skin biopsy specimen is the simplest and reliable test of acute GVHD.

Differential Diagnosis

- Viral exanthema
- Drug-induced maculopapular rash.

Management

Early diagnosis is the mainstay in the management of this fatal disorder and dermatologists may play a role in identifying this condition with the onset of the rash. Treatment of GVHD is the domain of hematologists and transplant surgeons. All patients having BMT/HSCT should receive prophylactic treatment with combination therapy of prednisolone, ciclosporin and methotrexate to prevent acute GVHD. In presence of erythroderma or SJS-like skin lesions, patient requires monitoring in a DICU. Early institution of low dose systemic steroid in patients presenting with grade I or grade II acute GVHD is associated with a better outcome.

In conclusion, some of the dermatological disorders present as acute emergency *per se*, e.g. Stevens-Johnson syndrome-toxic epidermal necrolysis, anaphylaxis, mucosal angioedema, extensive immunobullous disorders, severe type 2 reaction and acute neuritis in leprosy, etc. Other disorders like erythroderma of any etiology, acute urticaria and angioedema, infectious diseases, etc. may give rise to emergency situation during the course of the disease. Whenever a patient is admitted with crisis or potential to develop so, it is the clinician's duty to assess the risk, transfer the patient to ICU/DICU immediately and initiate the management protocol so that the valuable minutes are not wasted.

SUGGESTED FURTHER READING

1. Bas M, Hoffmann TK, Bier H, Kojda G. Increased C-reactive protein in ACE-inhibitor-induced angioedema. Br J Clin Pharmacol 2005;59:233–8.
2. Bonamigo RR, Razera F, Cartell A. Extensive skin necrosis following use of noradrenaline and dopamine. JEADV 2007;21:565–6.
3. Brady WJ, DeBehnke J, Crosby DL. Dermatological emergencies. Am J Emerg Med 1994;12:217–37.
4. Breathnach SM, Smith CH, Chalmers RJG, Hay RJ. Systemic therapy. In:Burns T, Breathnach S, Cox N, Griffiths C, editors. Rook's textbook of dermatology, 8th edition. Oxford: Wiley-Blackwell;2010. p-74.1–74.54.

5. Breathnach SM. Drug reactions. In:Burns T, Breathnach S, Cox N, Griffiths C, editors. Rook's textbook of dermatology, 8th edition. Oxford: Wiley-Blackwell;2010;p-75.1–75.178.
6. Breathnach SM. Erythema multiforme, Stevens-Johnson syndrome, Toxic epidermal necrolysis. In:Burns T, Breathnach S, Cox N, Griffiths C, editors. Rook's textbook of dermatology, 8th edition. Oxford: Wiley-Blackwell;2010. p-76.1–76.22.
7. Burns DA. Diseases caused by arthropods and other noxious animals. In:Burns T, Breathnach S, Cox N, Griffiths C, editors. Rook's textbook of dermatology, 8th edition. Oxford: Wiley-Blackwell;2010.p-38.1-38.62.
8. Burr JA. Efficacy of icabitant as treatment for ACE-inhibitor-induced angioedema in adults: a systematic review [Capstone project]. Oregon:Pacific University,2011. Available at http://commons.pacificu.edu/pa/235. Accessed on June 30th, 2012.
9. Caballero T, Farkas H, Bouillet L, Bowen T, Gompel A, Fagerberg G, et al. International consensus and practical guidelines on the gynecologic and obstetric management of female patients with hereditary angioedema caused by C1 inhibitor deficiency. J Allergy Clin Immunol 2012;129:308–20.
10. Cox NH, Coulson IH. Systemic diseases and the skin. In:Burns T, Breathnach S, Cox N, Griffiths C, editors. Rook's textbook of dermatology, 8th edition. Oxford: Wiley-Blackwell;2010. p-62.1-62.114.
11. Dunnill MGS, Handfield-Jones SE, Treacher D, McGibbon DH. Dermatology in the intensive care unit. Br J Dermatol 1995;132:226–35.
12. Ferrara JLM, Yanik G. Acute graft versus host disease:pathophysiology, risk factors, and prevention strategies. Clin Adv Hematol Oncol 2005;3:415–9.
13. Goldenberg NA, Manco-Johnson MJ. Protein C deficiency. Hemophilia 2008;14:1214–21.
14. Halstead SB. Dengue fever and dengue hemorrhagic fever. In: Kliegman RM, Behrman RE, Jenson HB, Stanton BF, editors. Nelson textbook of pediatrics, 18th edition. Philadelphia: Elsevier Saunders;2008.p-1412–15.
15. Hook EW, Handsfield HH. Gonococcal infections in the adult. In: Holmes KK, Sparling PF, Stamm WE, Piot P, Wasserheit JN, Corey L, et al, editors. Sexually transmitted diseases, 4th edition. New York: McGraw Hill;2008.p-627–45.
16. Inamadar AC, Palit A, Ragunatha S, Sampagavi VV, Deshmukh NS, Anitha B. Cutaneous loxoscelism. What's new in dermatology? 2008; 54:19–21.
17. Inamadar AC, Palit A. Drug hypersensitivity syndrome. In: Ghosh S, editor. Recent advances in dermatology. New Delhi: Jaypee Brothers Medical Publishers (P) Ltd;2007.p-129–41.
18. Jantschitsch C, Kinaciyan T, Manafi M, Safer M, Tanew A. Severe scombroid fish poisoning: an under recognized dermatologic emergency. J Am Acad Dermatol 2011;65:246–7.
19. Kaiber FL, Malucelli TO, Baroni ERV, Schafranski MD, Akamatsu HT, Schmidt CCF. Heparin-induced thrombocytopenia and warfarin-induced skin necrosis: a case report. An Bras Dermatol 2010;85:915–8.
20. Kanani A, Schellenberg R, Warrington R. Urticaria and angioedema. Allergy Asthma Clin Immunol 2011; 7(Suppl 1):S9.
21. Kar HK, Sharma P. Leprosy reactions. In: Kar HK, Kumar B, editors. IAL textbook of leprosy. New Delhi: Jaypee Brothers Medical Publishers (P) Ltd;2010. p-269-89.

22. Katsourakis A, Noussios G, Kapoutsis G, Chatzitheoklitos E. Low molecular weight heparin-induced skin necrosis: A case report. Case Report Med 2011; 2011:857391.
23. Kim EH, Lee SH, Byun SW, Kang HS, Koo DH, Park H-G, et al. Skin necrosis after a low-dose vasopressin infusion through a central venous catheter for treating septic shock. Korean J Intern Med 2006;21:287–90.
24. Kim H, Fischer D. Anaphylaxis. Allergy Asthma Clin Immunol 2011; 7(Suppl 1):S6.
25. Kloth N, Lane AS. ACE-inhibitor-induced angioedema: a case report and review of current management. Crit Care Resusc 2011;13:33–7.
26. Korniyenko A, Alviar CL, Cordova JP, Messerli FH. Visceral angioedema due to angiotensin-converting enzyme inhibitor therapy. Cleveland Clinic Journal of Medicine 2011;78:297–304.
27. Ladhani S, Garbash M. Staphylococcal skin infections in children. Rational drug therapy recommendations. Pediatr Drugs 2006;7:77–102.
28. Ladhani S, Joannou CL, Lochrie DP, Evans RW, Poston SM. Clinical, microbial and biochemical aspects of the exfoliative toxins causing staphylococcal scalded skin syndrome. Clin Microbiol Rev 1999;12:224–42.
29. Langhurst H, Cicardi M. Hereditary angio-oedema. Lancet 2012;379: 474–81.
30. Mielcarek M, Storer BE, Boeckh M, Carpenter PA, McDonald GB, Deeg HJ, et al. Initial therapy of acute graft-versus-host disease with low-dose prednisone does not compromise patient outcomes. Blood 2009;113:2888–94.
31. Mortimer PS, Burnand KG, Neumann HAM. Diseases of the veins and arteries: leg ulcers. In:Burns T, Breathnach S, Cox N, Griffiths C, editors. Rook's textbook of dermatology, 8th edn. Oxford: Wiley-Blackwell;2010. p-47.1-47.58.
32. Moss C, Shahidullah H. Naevi and other developmental defects. In:Burns T, Breathnach S, Cox N, Griffiths C, editors. Rook's textbook of dermatology, 8th edition. Oxford:Wiley-Blackwell;2010. p-18.1-18.108.
33. Mukasa Y, Craven N. Management of toxic epidermal necrolysis and related syndromes. Postgrad Med J 2008;84:60–66.
34. Nazarian RM, Van Cott EM, Zembowicz A, Duncan LM. Warfarin-induced skin necrosis. J Am Acad Dermatol 2009;61:325–32.
35. Palit A, Inamadar AC. Purpura fulminans in children: an update. In: Inamadar AC, Palit A, editors. Advances in pediatric dermatology, 1st edition. New Delhi: Jaypee Brothers Medical Publishers (P) Ltd; 2011. p-198–214.
36. Palit A, Ragunatha S. Nutritional deficiency disorders. In:Inamadar AC, Sacchidanand S, editors. Textbook of pediatric dermatology, 1st edition. New Delhi: Jaypee Brothers Medical Publishers (P) Ltd; 2009. p-198–214.
37. Rice PA, Handsfield HH. Arthritis associated with sexually transmitted diseases. In: Holmes KK, Sparling PF, Stamm WE, Piot P, Wasserheit JN, Corey L, et al, editors. Sexually transmitted diseases, 4th edition. New York: McGraw Hill;2008.p-1259–76.
38. Ross EA. Evolution of treatment strategies for calciphylaxis. Am J Nephrol 2011;34:460–7.
39. Rothe MJ, Bialy TL, Grant-Kels JM. Erythroderma. Dermatol Clin 2000;18: 405–15.
40. Rowley AH, Shulman ST. Kawasaki disease. In: Kliegman RM, Behrman RE, Jenson HB, Stanton BF, editors. Nelson textbook of pediatrics, 18th edition. Philadelphia: Elsevier Saunders;2008.p-1036–41.

41. Ruiz-Irastorza G, Crowther M, Branch W, Khamashta MA. Antiphospholipid syndrome. September 6, 2010. Available at www. thelancet.com, Accessed on June 12th, 2012.
42. Saigal R, Kansal A, Mittal M, Singh Y, Ram H. Antiphospholipid antibody syndrome. JAPI 2010;58:176–84.
43. Sarkany RPE, Breathnach SM, Morris AAM, Weissmann K, Flynn PD. Metabolic and nutritional disorders. In:Burns T, Breathnach S, Cox N, Griffiths C, editors. Rook's textbook of dermatology, 8th edition. Oxford: Wiley-Blackwell;2010. p-59.1-59.104.
44. Seetharam KA. Emerging infectious diseases. In: Inamadar AC, Palit A, editors. Advances in pediatric dermatology, 1st edition. New Delhi: Jaypee Brothers Medical Publishers (P) Ltd;2011. p-83–110.
45. Sexually transmitted diseases treatment guidelines, 2010.MMWR, December 17, 2010/Vol. 59/No.RR-12. Available at www.cdc.gov/mmwr. Accessed on 12th July, 2012.
46. Siberry GK, Dumler JS. Spotted fever group. Rickettsioses. In: Kliegman RM, Behrman RE, Jenson HB, Stanton BF, editors. Nelson textbook of pediatrics, 18th edition. Philadelphia: Elsevier Saunders;2008.p-1289–94.
47. Sontheimer RD, McCauliffe P. Lupus-specific skin disease. In: Wallace DJ, Hahn BH, editors. Dubois' Lupus erythematosus , 7th edition. Philadelphia: Lippincott Williams & Wilkins;2007.p-576–620.
48. Stevens DL, Bisno AL, Chambers HF, Everett ED, Dellinger P, Goldstein EJ, et al. Practice guidelines for the diagnosis and management of skin and soft-tissue infections. Clin Infect Dis 2005;41:1373–1406.
49. White B, Smith OP. Infectious purpura fulminans; diagnosis and treatment. Br J Haematol 1999;104:202–7.
50. Wojnarowska F, Venning VA. Immunobullous diseases. In:Burns T, Breathnach S, Cox N, Griffiths C, editors. Rook's textbook of dermatology, 8th edition. Oxford:Wiley-Blackwell;2010. p-40.1-40.62.
51. Wolf R, Orion E, Marcos B, Matz H. Life-threatening acute adverse cutaneous drug reactions. Clin Dermatol 2005;23:171–81.
52. Wolkenstein P, Revuz J. Toxic epidermal necrolysis. Dermatol Clin 2000; 18:485–95.
53. Woods CR. Neisseria meningitides (Meningococcus). In: Kliegman RM, Behrman RE, Jenson HB, Stanton BF, editors. Nelson textbook of pediatrics, 18th edition. Philadelphia: Elsevier Saunders;2008.p-1164–69.
54. Zajicek R, Pintar D, Broz L, Suca H, Königova R. Toxic epidermal necrolysis and Stevens-Johnson syndrome at the Prague burn centre 1998–2008. JEADV 2012;26:639–43.

chapter 3

Fluid, Electrolyte and Nutrition Therapy in Dermatological Emergencies

Ragunatha S, Kumar GV

- Body fluid compartments
- Fluid, electrolyte disturbances and protein loss in acute skin failure
- Fluid, electrolyte and nutritional therapy in dermatological emergencies
- Fluid resuscitation in patients with TEN
- Fluid and electrolyte therapy in erythroderma
- Nutritional supplementation in patients with dermatological emergencies

INTRODUCTION

Skin is the largest organ of body performing various protective, synthetic and metabolic functions, which are essential for maintaining homeostasis of body. Loss of cutaneous barrier usually increases the risk of infection with various microorganisms. If there is extensive denudation of skin (e.g. in erythroderma/Stevens-Johnson syndrome (SJS)-Toxic epidermal necrolysis (TEN)/immunobullous and mechanobullous disorders), significant fluid and electrolyte deficiency may occur due to increased transepidermal water loss (TEWL) with or without solutes. The loss of barrier function along with inability to maintain core body temperature results in a state of acute skin failure. Adequate fluid, electrolyte and nutritional replacements are essential for successful therapeutic outcome in a patient with acute skin failure. It depends upon the nature of the underlying cutaneous disease and composition of the fluid lost. Understanding of composition and distribution of body fluids and solutes helps in judicious therapeutic use of fluid and electrolytes. Studies on estimation of fluid and electrolyte loss in patients with acute skin failure and related management are very limited. Therefore, the guidelines used in burn patients for management of fluid, electrolyte and nutrition are extrapolated for the treatment of patients with toxic epidermal necrolysis.

BODY FLUID COMPARTMENTS

Water constitutes approximately 50% of the body weight in women and 60% in men. Total body water is distributed into two major compartments, intracellular fluid (ICF) and extracellular fluid (ECF). ICF constitutes 55 to 75% and the ECF constitutes 25 to 45% of total body water. Extracellular fluid is further divided into intravascular space and extravascular space in a ratio of 1:3 (**Figure 3.1**).

The solute or particle concentration of a fluid determines its osmolality. The osmotic equilibrium where extracellular fluid osmolality is equal to that of intracellular fluid is achieved by movement of water across the cell membrane. The major ECF particles are Na^+, Cl^- and HCO_3^-, whereas K^+, adenosine triphosphate, creatinine phosphate and phospholipids are major ICF particles. The number of intracellular particles remains constant as these are required for normal cell function. Therefore, the changes in ICF osmolality are due to changes in ICF water content. For normal functioning of cells, maintenance of osmotic equilibrium is important. To maintain this steady state, water intake must be equal to water excretion.

Normally, in addition to mandatory water loss through the kidneys and gastrointestinal system, water is evaporated from the skin and respiratory tract. The latter two are not measured usually and hence termed as insensible water loss (IWL). Transepidermal water loss contributes 70% of this insensible water loss. Therefore, the fluid and electrolyte loss that occur in acute skin failure results in hemodynamic and metabolic changes and systemic organ dysfunction.

FLUID, ELECTROLYTE DISTURBANCES AND PROTEIN LOSS IN ACUTE SKIN FAILURE

There is significant loss of fluid and electrolytes through the skin in two clinical settings;
- In the first, transepidermal water loss (TEWL) occurs through erythrodermic skin leading to hypernatremic dehydration. It is seen in

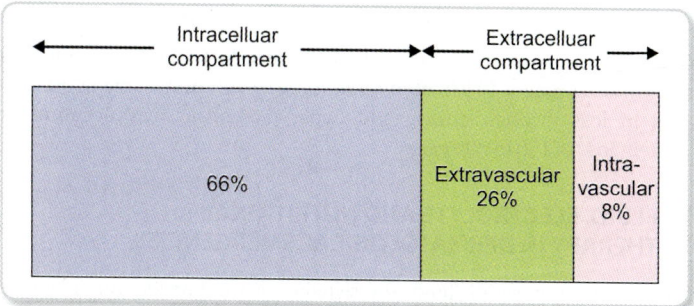

Figure 3.1: Approximate distribution of total body water

dermatoses presenting as diffuse scaling, e.g. congenital ichthyoses, psoriasis, atopic dermatitis, drug reactions, etc.
- In the second, both water and electrolytes are lost through eroded skin. It is seen in autoimmune blistering disorders and SJS-TEN.

In adult patients with toxic epidermal necrolysis involving >50% of total body surface area (TBSA), the daily fluid loss exceeds 3 to 4 liters. Following is the blister fluid content in autoimmune bullous disorders and TEN;

> The blister fluid of autoimmune bullous disorders and TEN contains approximately:
> - 120–150 mmol/L of Na^+
> - 100 mmol/L of Cl^-
> - 5–10 mmol/L of K^+
> - 40 g/L of protein

In children with ichthyosis, the total body transepidermal water loss ranges from 746 ± 468 ml/day, depending upon the severity and genetic heterogeneity (mean basal TEWL of 39.6 ± 20.6 ml/m²/hour, as compared to upper limit of normal 8.7 ml/m²/hour). This is in contrast to 209 ml/day seen in age-matched children with competent skin barrier. An estimation of TEWL from normal and abnormal skin of a collodion baby using evaporimeter at day 4 demonstrated a loss of 18 ± 2 g/m²/hour and 112 ± 2 g/m²/hour of water respectively, at room temperature of 27°C and relative humidity of 25%. It reduces significantly, in parallel with the clinical improvement of the skin at day 30 to 5.5 ± 2 g/m²/hour and 16 ± 2 g/m²/hour respectively, at room temperature of 23⁰C and relative humidity of 37%.

Apart from fluid and electrolytes, major nutrients like proteins are also lost. The patients with diffuse scaling are more predisposed to protein loss through exfoliation. Normal daily exfoliated material from skin amounts to 500 to 1000 mg; in acute skin failure, there is a 9-fold increase in this.

> Diffuse scaling leads to protein loss of approximately 20–30 g/m² BSA/day.

The blister fluid of autoimmune bullous disorders and toxic epidermal necrolysis contains 40 g/L of protein. In these conditions, the combined protein loss through oozing and hyper-catabolism may account for protein loss of 150 to 200 g/day.

FLUID, ELECTROLYTE AND NUTRITIONAL THERAPY IN DERMATOLOGICAL EMERGENCIES

The main purpose of fluid resuscitation is to provide an adequate intravascular volume to perfuse essential internal viscera and peripheral tissues. The purpose of fluid and electrolyte therapy includes:

- Restoration of losses that have already occurred,
- Replacement of ongoing losses, and
- Maintenance of fluid.

Decision on fluid resuscitation depends upon:
- Composition of the fluid lost,
- Severity of the dehydration,
- Underlying disease, and
- Age of the patient.

The infants and younger children have a larger daily turnover of water relative to total body water and large extracellular fluid space, whereas the neonates have high body surface area to weight ratio and functionally immature kidneys. All these factors predispose the children to a greater risk of fluid and electrolyte imbalance than adults.

FLUID RESUSCITATION IN PATIENTS WITH TEN

The epidermal denudation that occurs at the level of dermo-epidermal junction in TEN resembles partial thickness or second degree superficial burns. Involvement of >10% of TBSA in children and >15% of TBSA in adults indicates requirement of intravenous fluid resuscitation. However, in patients with toxic epidermal necrolysis the loss of fluid and electrolytes is far lower than what is seen in burns.

> In TEN fluid and electrolyte loss is lower than in burns, because of:
> - Absence of thermal effects,
> - Moderate papillary edema, and
> - Sparing of reticular dermis.

Hence, in toxic epidermal necrolysis the fluid therapy need not be as aggressive as in burns. The resuscitation fluid requirement is 2/3rd to 3/4th of that of burns covering the same area.

Assessment of Body Surface Area Involved

Various methods are followed to assess the extent of the body surface area involved. 'Rule of nine' is used for immediate assessment and it gives approximate values (**Figure 3.2**). This method should not be used in children less than 15 years of age. A more accurate method is, drawing the involved area on Lund-Browder Chart. The size of the palm of the patient including fingers corresponds to 1% of total body surface area. This method of assessment is useful only in small area of burns.

Calculation of Replacement Fluid (First 24 Hours)

The calculation of replacement fluid during first 24 hours from the time of injury is similar to that of burns. The *Parkland formula* which is based on

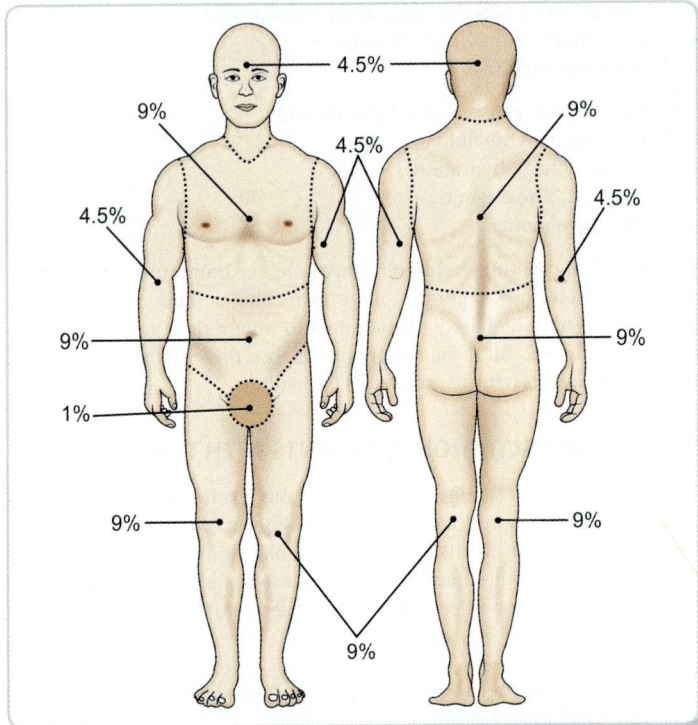

Figure 3.2: 'Rule of nine' for calculation of body surface area (http://www.emedicinehealth.com/burn_percentage_in_adults_rule_of_nine/article_em.htm)

crystalloids is commonly used to calculate resuscitation fluid volume for the first 24 hours from the time of injury.

> *Parkland formula:* Resuscitation volume = 4 ml × total body weight × % of epidermolytic body surface involved.

In children weighing < 40 kg, additional maintenance fluid is added to the initial resuscitation volume. Half of the calculated volume is administered in first 8 hours and remaining half in subsequent 16 hours.

Calculation of Maintenance Fluid and Ongoing Evaporative Fluid Loss

After initial 24 hours, the fluid therapy includes *'maintenance fluid'* and *'ongoing evaporative water loss'* from the eroded skin. The volume of maintenance fluid is determined from metabolic rate. Accordingly, 100 ml of exogenous water is required for 100 kcal of energy metabolized.

The caloric expenditure and maintenance fluid requirement is estimated as follows:

- 100 ml/kg/day for first 10 kg (1000 ml),
- 50 ml/kg/day for next 10 kg (1000 ml+500 ml), and
- 20 ml/kg/day above 20 kg (1500 ml+20 ml/kg).

The evaporative loss of fluid is calculated by using following formulas:

- Insensible water loss (IWL) = (125 + % TBSA involved) × TBSA (m²)
- Evaporative water loss (through eroded skin in children) = (125 + % TBSA involved) × TBSA (m²)

Choice of Fluid

The main aim of fluid therapy during first 24 hours is rapid restoration of intravascular volume. Commonly used fluid for replacement during first 24 hour is Ringer's lactate. In infants and younger children who are more prone to develop hypernatremia and lactic acidosis, 0.33% saline is preferred instead of Ringer's lactate.

The parenteral solution for maintenance therapy should contain 25 to 30 mEq/L of Na^+ and Cl^-, 20 mEq/L of K^+, and 5% dextrose.

The evaporative loss is replaced preferably with free water. However, 5% dextrose in 0.2% saline is used to prevent water intoxication and electrolyte imbalance.

Colloidal resuscitation with 5% human albumin in normal saline is recommended if the BSA involved is > 40%, as the hyper-catabolic state and movement of protein into extravascular space result in significant amount of protein loss. It is estimated as 0.3–0.4 ml/kg×% of BSA involved, administered over 6 to 8 hours. Though colloids rapidly restore the intravascular volume, these are not preferred during the first 24 hours after injury because of presence of capillary leak. Hence, colloid resuscitation is recommended only after 24 hours.

Route of Administration

Generally, oral resuscitation is preferred. However, if total body surface area involved is >10% in children and >15% in adults, intravenous administration of fluid is recommended. Oral fluid can be started within 24 hours if the patient is not in severe shock. Initially, 1/4th of the daily requirement is given orally. Gradually oral intake is increased and intravenous fluid is decreased accordingly.

Monitoring

The estimation of fluid volume by resuscitation formulas gives only a rough guide to the fluid therapy. Frequent clinical and laboratory monitoring is essential for successful fluid and electrolyte resuscitation. Hydration status of the patient can be checked at baseline and thereafter at intervals by checking peripheral skin turgor, urine output and specific gravity of urine. The main aim of resuscitation is to maintain normal urine output (0.5–1 ml/kg/hour), blood pressure, serum sodium and heart rate. In children capillary filling time is also monitored. More accurate invasive monitoring techniques like central venous pressure and pulmonary wedge pressure are not recommended to avoid the risk of invasive sepsis.

Measurement of urine output is considered as the surrogate marker of successful fluid therapy. Urine output ≤ 1/3rd of the predicted value over two consecutive hours should prompt the increase in intravenous fluid administration. Similarly, if it is more than predicted value, the intravenous fluid needs to be decreased. In such situations, the conservative approach is to increase or decrease intravenous fluid rate by 20%/hour. Some recommend increase in intravenous fluid by 50%, if urine output is <1 ml/kg/hour and decrease the rate of infusion if urine output is > 2 ml/kg/hour.

FLUID AND ELECTROLYTE THERAPY IN ERYTHRODERMA

The dermatological conditions characterized by diffuse scaling and erythema result in increased TEWL. Solute free loss of water leads to hypernatremic dehydration especially in children. In infants and young children the estimation of severity of volume contraction on the basis of common clinical signs is difficult (**Table 3.1**). In addition, inability of these children to drink water on their own in response to hypernatremia associated thirst results in severe hypernatremic dehydration. As in other types of dehydration, rapid restoration of intravascular volume is achieved by infusion of Ringer's lactate or normal saline (10–20 ml/kg/hour), administered over 1 to 2 hours. In infants, particularly in premature

Table 3.1: Clinical signs of severity of dehydration in infants and children

1.	Mild dehydration	• Loss of body weight by 3–5% • Minimal clinical signs • Decreased urination
2.	Moderate dehydration	• Loss of body weight by 6–10% • Tenting of skin • Lethargy • Sunken eyes
3.	Severe dehydration	• Loss of body weight by 11–15% • Hypotension • Tachypnea • Tachycardia • Oliguria • Altered sensorium

infants normal saline is preferred. The deficit calculated based on serum sodium should be replaced over 48 to 72 hours.

> Water deficit = (plasma Na⁺ concentration − 140 ÷ 140) × total body water [in hypernatremia total body water is 50% (men) and 40% (women) of lean body weight]

The fluid should be administered slowly to prevent brain cell injury from intracellular edema that occurs during the process of rehydration. Therefore, careful evaluation of the patient and serum sodium is important. During the slow rehydration, the therapy should provide deficit fluid, standard maintenance fluid and ongoing losses. The parenteral solution used for maintenance therapy (5% dextrose in 0.2% saline) is preferred. The serum sodium should fall by 0.4 to 0.8 mEq/L/hour or 10 to 12 mEq/L/day. A rapid fall in serum sodium indicates overzealous replacement, indicating the need for slowing of rate of rehydration. Similarly, increase in serum sodium indicates inadequate replacement indicating need to increase the rate of rehydration.

NUTRITIONAL SUPPLEMENTATION IN PATIENTS WITH DERMATOLOGICAL EMERGENCIES

Similar to fluid and electrolyte therapy, nutritional supplementation in patients with toxic epidermal necrolysis is similar to that of patients with burns with same BSA involvement. In patients with large BSA involvement, the hyper-metabolic state, fluid loss, and sepsis contributes to 50% increase in protein metabolism and energy expenditure. Adults with >15% and children with >10% of BSA involvement have an increased nutritional requirement.

The TEWL is always accompanied by heat loss at the rate of 0.58 kcal/ml. The total calorie loss from daily TEWL in pediatric patients with ichthyosis ranges from 84 to 1015 kcal (21 ± 9.8 kcal/kg/day with a mean of 433 ± 272 kcal/day) in contrast to 41 to 132 kcal/day seen in age-matched normal children. Therefore, aggressive nutrition supplementation should be started with the following aims:

- To minimize the catabolism of proteins
- To provide proteins required for healing of skin lesions
- To ensure rapid growth of the child.

The feeding should be started within 6 hours of the injury if gastrointestinal functions are intact. Enteral feeding is preferred as it has the advantage of preserving gastrointestinal integrity and decreasing the incidence of bacterial transmigration across the gut. Enteral feeding may be carried out by 'oral sip feeding' or 'tube feeding' through Ryle's tube.

Severely ill patients may have impaired gastric emptying. Hence, the enteral feeding is initially started with 1/4th of the desired volume, which is gradually increased at a rate of 5 ml/hour. The residual gastric volume should be checked by periodic aspiration and feeding is stopped if it is more than 50 ml.

Critically ill patients undergoing enteral feeding are prone to develop feeding related complications as follows:

- More than 30% patients develop diarrhea, bloating and vomiting.
- Inadvertent feeding/positioning of the patient may lead to aspiration.

In children with TEN involving <20% of BSA, the gastrointestinal activity returns to normal within 72 hours. In extensive involvement, paralytic ileus persists for > 5 to 6 days. Various formulas have been used for calculation of protein and caloric requirements (**Table 3.2**).

For enteral feeding, isodense formulas that give 100 kcal/100 ml are preferred and are well-tolerated. Caloric value of some common food items are as follows:
- Milk 100 ml = 60 kcal
- Sugar 1 tsp = 20 kcal
- Cereals 1.5 tsp = 20 kcal
- Cereal pulse mix (1tsp SAT mix) = 20 kcal

Based on caloric values of these food items, various kitchen-based isodense enteral feeding are prepared. Following are some of the examples:
- SAT mix, a precooked ready to mix cereal pulse sugar mixture containing rice, wheat, black gram and sugar in the ratio of 1:1:1:2 can be used with milk. Two table spoon of SAT mix in ½ glass milk (100 ml) gives 100 kcal/100 ml. SAT mix 100 g supplies 308 kcal and 8 g protein.
- High energy milk containing ½ glass milk, 1 tsp sugar and ½ tsp oil.
- Cereal milk containing ½ glass milk, 1 tsp sugar and 1.5 tsp cereal flour.
- Fruit juice containing 1 orange, 2 tsp sugar and water up to 100 ml.
- Egg flip containing 1 egg, 2 tsp sugar and ¾ glass milk.

Table 3.2: Protein and calorie requirement recommended for patients with TEN

Calorie	Protein
Sutherland formula: Children: 60 kcal/kg + 35 kcal/% BSA involved Adults: 60 kcal/kg + 35 kcal/% BSA involved	*Davies formula:* Children: 3 g/kg + 1 g/% BSA involved Adults: 1 g/kg + 3 g/% BSA involved
Modified Harris-Benedict formula: 0–12 months: 2100 kcal/m^2 + 1000 kcal/m^2 TBSA involved 1–11 years: 1800 kcal/m^2 + 1300 kcal/m^2 TBSA involved 12 years and older: 1500 kcal/m^2 + 1500 kcal/m^2 TBSA involved	

Enteral feeding preparations are also available commercially in Indian market *viz.* Pepti-2000, Bonvit, Recupex, ToCal, Renocare, Ten-o-Lip LF (Lactose free), Glutameal, Promilac, Protal M, Nusobee and Pediasure.

The food for the patients in DICU must be kept in sealed container, preferably at – 4°C. Canned foods are discarded once the container is open.

In addition to protein and energy, daily supplementation of vitamins, minerals and trace elements are also to be provided. Milk, fruit juice and honey constitute important source of potassium.

A comprehensive daily dietary schedule for patients with SJS-TEN has been recommended in 'Proposed IADVL consensus guidelines for management of SJS-TEN' which may be followed for this group of patients.

In conclusion, fluid, electrolyte and nutrition therapy is the crux of management of the patients with dermatological emergency. The DICU team must be conversant with maintenance of intake-output chart, calculation of oral/IV fluid, electrolyte requirement and recognize the clinical signs of deficit in a critically ill patient. Nutritional supplement is another important aspect of management of these patients. Though the dermatologists are conversant with dietary protocol of patients with acute skin failure, inclusion of a dietician in the DICU team is appropriate to carry out this function.

SUGGESTED FURTHER READING

1. Atiyeh BS, Dham R, Yassin MF, El-Musa KA. Treatment of toxic epidermal necrolysis with moisture—retentive ointment: A case report and review of the literature. Dermatol Surg 2003;29:185–8.
2. Buyse L, Graves C, Marks R, Wijeyesekera K, Alfaham M, Finlay AY. Collodion baby dehydration: the danger of high transepidermal water loss. Br J Dermatol 1993;129:86–8.
3. Chawla D, Agarwal R, Deorari AK, Paul VK. Fluid and Electrolyte management in term and preterm neonates. Indian J Pediatr 2008;75:255-9.
4. Elizebeth KE. Nutrition in health and illness. In: Gupte S, editor. Textbook of pediatric nutrition. New Delhi: PeePee Publishers and Distributors (P) Ltd; 2006.p-351-57.
5. Finkelstein JL, Schwartz SB, Madden MR, Marano MA, Goodwin CW. Pediatric burns. An overview. Pediatr Clin Nor Am 1992; 39: 1145–64.
6. Fromowitz JS, Ramos-Caro FS, Flowers FP. Practical guidelines for the management of toxic epidermal necrolysis and Stevens–Johnson syndrome. Int J Dermatol 2007;46:1092–4.
7. Gerdts B, Vloemans AFPM, Kreis RW. Toxic epidermal necrolysis; 15 years' experience in a Dutch burns centre. J Eur Acad Dermatol Venereol 2007;21:781–8.
8. Inamadar AC, Palit A. Acute skin failure: Concept, causes, consequences and care. Indian J Dermatol Venereol Leprol 2005;71:379–85.

9. Kimgai-Asadi A, Freedberg IM. Exfoliative dermatitis. In: Freedberg IM, Eisen AZ, Wolff K, Austen KF, Goldsmith LA, Katz SI, editors. Fitzpatrick's Dermatology in General Medicine, 6th edition. New York: McGraw-Hill; 2003.p-436-41.
10. MacFie J. Nutrition and fluid therapy. In: Williams NS, Bulstrode CJK, O'Connell PR, editors. Bailey & Love's short practice of surgery, 25th edition. London:Hodder Arnold; 2008.p-222-33.
11. Mosowtz DG, Fowler AJ, Heyman MB, Cohen SP, Crumrine D, Elias PM. Pathophysiologic basis for growth failure in children with ichthyosis: an evaluation of cutaneous ultrastructure, epidermal permeability, barrier function, and energy expenditure. J Pediatr 2004;145:82–92.
12. Ragunatha S, Inamadar AC. Neonatal dermatological emergencies. Indian J Dermatol Venereol Leprol 2010;76:328–40.
13. Revuz J, Roujeau JC, Guillaume JC, Penso D, Touraine R. Treatment of toxic epidermal necrolysis. Creteil's experience. Arch Dermatol 1987; 123:1156–8.
14. Richards WT, Mozingo DW. Burn injury: thermal and electrical. In: Gabrielli A, Layon AJ, Yu M, editors. Civett, Teylor and Kirby's Critical Care, 4th edItion. Philadelphia: Lippincott Williams and Wilkins; 2009. p-1313–24.
15. Roujeau JC, Revuz J. Intensive care in dermatology. In: Champion RH, Pye RJ, editors. Recent advances in dermatology, Vol 8. Edinburgh: Churchill Livinstone; 1990.p-85-100.
16. Sharma VK, Jerajani HR, Srinivas CR, Valia A, Khandpur S. Proposed IADVL consensus guidelines 2006: Management of Stevens-Johnson syndrome (SJS) and toxic epidermal necrolysis (TEN). IADVL News 2006;2(1):85–93.
17. Siegel NS, Lattazi WE. Fluid and electrolyte therapy in children. In: Arieff AI, DeFronzo RA, editors. Fluid, electrolyte and acid-base disorders, 1st edition. New York: Churchill Livingstone; 1985.p-1211-30.
18. Singer GG, Brenner BM. Fluid and electrolyte disturbances. In: Braunwald E, Fauci AS, Kasper DL, Hauser SL, Longo DL, Jameson JL, editors. Harrison's principles in Internal Medicine, 15th edition. New York: McGraw-Hill; 2001.p-271–83.
19. Tyler M, Ghosh S. Burns. In: William NS, Bulstrode CJK, O'Connell PR, editors. Bailey and Love's Short Practice of Surgery, 25th edition. London: Hodder Arnold; 2008.p-378-93.
20. Yurt RW, Howell JD, Greenwald BM. Burns, electrical injury and smoke inhalation. In: Helfaer MA, Nichols DG, editors. Roger's Handbook of pediatric intensive care, 4th edition. New Delhi: Lippincott Williams and Wilkins; 2009.p-59-66.

chapter 4

Procedures and Techniques in Dermatological Emergencies

Nazeer Ahmed K

- Vital signs and monitoring
- Universal precautions
- Procedures and maneuvers
- Vascular access
- Airway access/Maintenance
- Nasogastric access
- Transurethral catheterization
- Cardiopulmonary resuscitation

INTRODUCTION

Care of patients in dermatological intensive care unit (DICU) need both interventions and monitoring related to vascular access, airway management and cardiopulmonary resuscitation. The ability to carry out these interventions is an essential skill in the field of medicine and should be learnt and mastered by all physicians including dermatologists. Although these procedures may appear simple when performed by an expert, it is in fact a difficult skill which requires considerable practice to achieve perfection. Evaluation of patient's vital parameters is essential before attempting any emergency procedure.

VITAL SIGNS AND MONITORING

Major physiological parameters available for evaluation of cardiopulmonary status are respiratory rate, pulse rate, blood pressure and temperature. These are simple, basic and noninvasive methods of monitoring the critically ill patients.

Respiratory Rate

The respiratory rate (RR) is the number of inspirations in full one minute. The normal RR in adults is about 14 to 16 breaths/minute and it decreases with age. RR increases in disease states associated with hyperthermia, hypoxia, metabolic acidosis, shock and stress. Decreased RR is observed with anemia, hypoglycemia, hypothermia and metabolic alkalosis. It is measured by manual counting or through monitor.

Pulse

The volume of blood ejected by the heart/minute is countable as pulse. Pulse is counted either by palpation or auscultation for one minute duration and the rate is documented. Normal pulse rate in a healthy individual varies from 60 to 90 beats/minute. Physiologically, pulse rate varies with age, body temperature, and level of anxiety. If continuous monitoring is necessary, pulse oximeter and electrocardiography (ECG) are the best options. If pulse rate is < 50 beats/minute, it is termed as bradycardia. In disease states it always indicates cardiac depression and advanced respiratory failure. Pulse rate of >100 beats/minute is termed as tachycardia. It may denote volume loss, hypoxia, fever, or fear/anxiety.

Blood Pressure

Blood pressure (BP) is the measure of the homeostatic relationship between cardiac output and the peripheral vascular resistance. It is affected by cardiac output, vasomotor tone and volume status of the patient. Perfusion to vital organs like heart, brain, kidney and liver is pressure dependent. The use of conventional sphygmomanometer for recording BP is simple and reliable. Systolic BP of < 80-90 mm Hg is indicative of hypotension and it may be a feature of shock.

Temperature

Recording body temperature is a routine part of initial vital sign assessment. Abnormal temperature may be a manifestation of an infectious, inflammatory or malignant disease. It may be reflective of altered metabolism or deranged thermoregulation as found in widespread loss of skin (acute skin failure).

In critically ill patients admitted in DICU, these parameters can be recorded through a multi- parameter monitor (**Figure 4.1A**). Pulse oximeter may be used to estimate the oxygen saturation of patient's blood (**Figure 4.1B**).

■ UNIVERSAL PRECAUTIONS

Universal precautions must be practiced for all patient contacts that expose the health care workers (HCW) to blood/blood contaminated body fluids. The potential for contact with a patient's blood or body fluids while performing emergency procedures increases with the inexperience of the HCW. Gloves, gowns, plastic aprons and eye shields must be worn while handling the high risk body fluids. Handwashing is the single most essential strategy for preventing transmission of various infections.

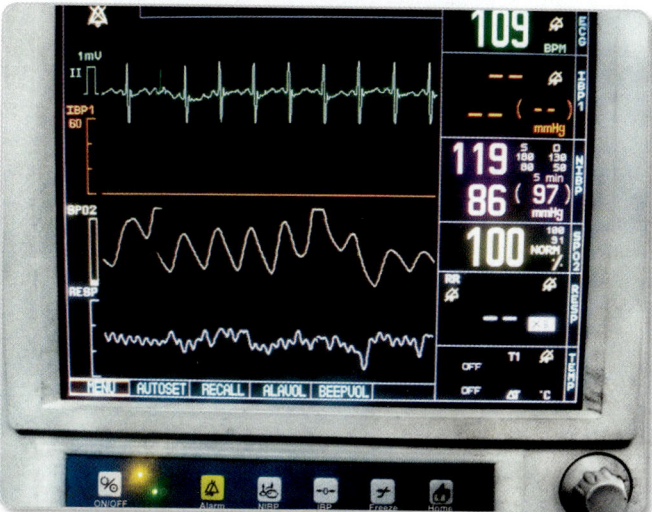

Figure 4.1A: Multi-parameter monitor showing oxygen saturation, heart rate, ECG and noninvasive blood pressure (NIBP)

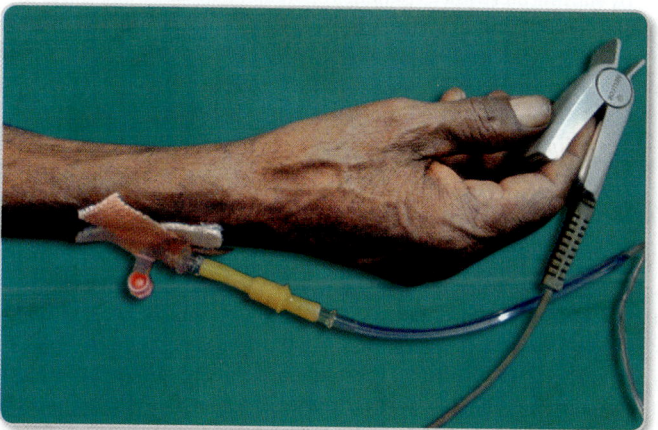

Figure 4.1B: Pulse oximeter probe attached to finger

PROCEDURES AND MANEUVERS

Following is the list of procedures or maneuvers which all medical professional including dermatologists must be conversant with;
- Vascular access
- Airway access
- Nasogastric access

- Urinary catheterization
- Cardiopulmonary resuscitation.

Universal precautions must be practiced strictly while performing these procedures and handling any patient in the critical care unit.

VASCULAR ACCESS

Management of critically ill patients in DICU needs insertion of one or more cannula to the vascular system for both monitoring and interventions. The art and craft of establishing vascular access has been emphasized here and some guidelines for insertion of vascular catheters and common percutaneous access routes have been described briefly. It is a skill to be mastered at the bedside.

Indications

- Blood sampling, volume resuscitation and administration of intravenous (IV) medications.
- Monitoring of fluid status.
- Total parenteral nutrition (TPN).
- Hemodialysis.

By starting an IV line, a patient's circulatory system is accessed, which enables a physician to draw sample of blood for investigations as well as to infuse IV fluids and medications. IV access is essential to manage all critically ill patients; some may require IV access in anticipation of future potential problems, when administration of fluid and/or drugs may be necessary for resuscitation.

Peripheral Venous Access

Sites for Peripheral Lines

Generally peripheral IV lines are initiated at the most distal site that is available and appropriate for this purpose. This allows cannulation of a more proximal site if initial attempt fails. If a proximal vein is punctured ineffectively, and thereafter IV channel is started at a distal site, there may be fluid leak from the injured proximal vessel. Following are the sites where peripheral venous lines may be set up:

- Dorsum of hand
- Forearm
- Antecubital fossa
- Dorsum of foot
- Saphenous vein
- External jugular veins
- Scalp veins.

Procedures and Techniques in Dermatological Emergencies

Figure 4.2 shows sites of peripheral venous access on dorsum of hand.

Equipment: Following are necessary for peripheral venous access:
- Appropriate size IV cannula, ranging from 14-24 G.
- Non-latex tourniquet.
- Swab soaked in alcohol/other cleanser.
- Sterile 2"x 2" gauze piece.
- Adhesive tape.
- IV fluid container with transfusion set.

Figure 4.3 shows the basic equipments necessary for peripheral venous access.

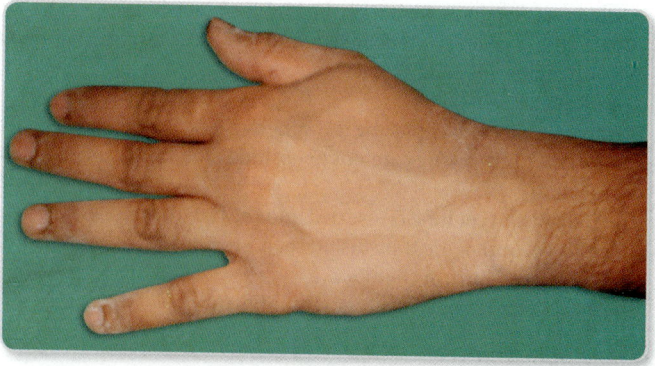

Figure 4.2: Sites of peripheral venous access on dorsum of hand

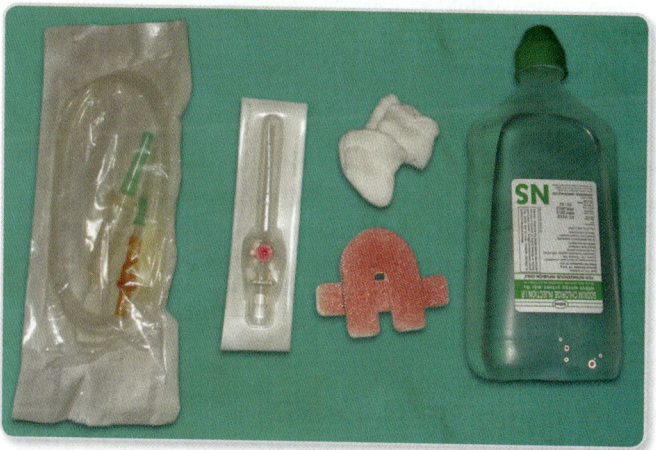

Figure 4.3: Basic equipments necessary for peripheral venous access (from left to right: IV transfusion set, IV cannula, swab soaked in alcohol, adhesive tape, IV fluid bottle)

Procedure
- Universal precautions to be adopted.
- Tourniquet is applied to the arm/leg above the site where IV cannulation has been planned.
- The vein is visualized and palpated.
- The site is cleaned with an antiseptic swab.
- The target vein is stabilized and counter tension applied to the skin.
- The stylet is pricked through the skin at an oblique angle and as it is advanced through the vein, the angle is reduced.
- The "flash back" is observed as blood slowly fills its chamber.
- The needle is advanced approximately 1 cm further into the vein.
- Holding the end of the catheter with thumb and index finger, only the needle is pulled back 1 cm with the middle finger.
- Slowly the catheter is advanced into the vein while maintaining tension on the vein and skin.
- Tourniquet is removed.
- Catheter is secured by placing the adhesive tape over the lower half of the catheter hub taking care not to occlude the transfusion set tubing connection.
- The transfusion set tube is inserted into the hub of the catheter.
- The roller clamp of the transfusion set is opened and observed for the fluid filling up the drip chamber.
- The fluid drop is adjusted as per requirement.

Complications
Following complications may arise following peripheral venous access:
- Extravasation of fluid
- Venous air embolism
- Infection at the site
- Thrombophlebitis.

Venesection
Though it is not performed routinely, it can be done in case of severe toxic epidermal necrolysis (TEN) or extensive immunobullous diseases where insertion of central line is not possible. Distal saphenous vein is an ideal site for venous cut down because of its consistent location and non-proximity with important structures.

Equipments for Venesection
Venesection tray should be equipped with the following:
- Sterile drapes
- Sterile gauze (4" × 4")

- Needles and syringes
- Scalpel blade (No 11 or 15)
- Curved Kelly hemostat
- Iris scissors
- Venesection catheter
- Vein introducer or hemostat
- Silk suture (3-0, 4-0)
- Cutting needle and needle holder

Procedure

Classical distal saphenous vein cut down is described below:
- Patient is made to rest in supine position, legs laterally rotated, so that medial aspect of distal leg and ankle faces upward. The leg is immobilized and placed on a padded board.
- Great saphenous vein is identified in front of medial malleolus.
- Sterile skin preparation and draping is done.
- Skin is infiltrated with 2% lignocaine injection with due care not to puncture the vein inadvertently.
- A transverse incision is made with No. 10 scalpel blade (patient's one finger's breadth superior and one finger's breadth anterior to medial malleolus, extending up to the anterior border of tibia).
- Saphenous vein is isolated on tibial surface using a curved hemostat.
- Two loops of 3-0 silk suture is passed under the vein, long enough to provide traction on the vein. The distal loop is used to ligate the vein to achieve a bloodless field. The proximal loop is used to pull the vein for stabilization.
- Venotomy is done using an iris scissors. The site is kept open with a hemostat/vein introducer and the catheter is advanced through the gap for 5 to 6 cm. It is correctly placed with a twisting motion and flushed with saline solution. As the catheter is long with small lumen blood reflux to it may be minimal/absent.
- The proximal loop is tied around the vein with catheter inside, taking care not to occlude it.
- The wound is closed with 4-0 silk and an additional suture is placed to secure the catheter through the skin. Appropriate dressing with antibiotic ointment is put to cover the wound.
- Catheter is closely checked for patency during every rounds.

Central Venous Catheterization (CVC)

Central venous catheter play an important role in the management of critically ill patients serving as a reliable vascular access. Intensivists usually insert CVC in large veins such as internal jugular vein, subclavian vein and femoral vein.

Indications

- For venous access when peripheral vein cannulation is not possible because of impaired skin integrity, as in erythroderma, SJS-TEN and extensive immunobullous disorders.
- Monitoring of body hydration status and cardiac chamber pressures.
- Administration of irritant medications or vasoactive substances.
- Total parenteral nutrition.

Sites

Following are the sites for central venous access:
- Antecubital vein
- Internal jugular vein (IJV)
- Femoral vein
- Subclavian vein.

Procedure

There are various sites through which central venous compartment can be accessed. But for convenience and simplicity right IJV approach has been described here:
- The patient is placed in a 15° Trendelenburg position and the head is turned to the contralateral side.
- Site: The triangle formed by the two bellies of the sterno-cleidomastoid muscle and the clavicle. (**Figure 4.4**).
- Necessary aseptic precautions taken.

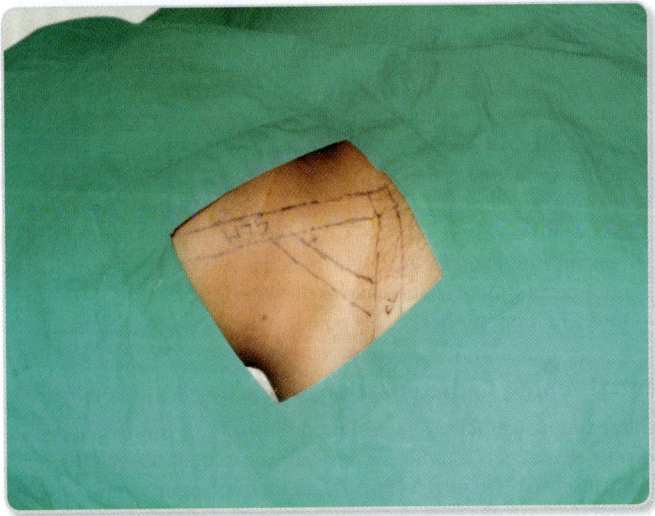

Figure 4.4: The triangle through which internal jugular vein is accessed for central venous catheterization (CL = clavicle, SCM = sternocleidomastoid muscle)

- Catheter insertion site is infiltrated with local anesthetic.
- Skin is punctured with a 22 gauge needle with an attached syringe at the apex of the triangle. The internal carotid artery pulsation is usually felt 1 to 2 cm medial to this point.
- The finder needle is directed at 45° angle towards the ipsilateral nipple with constant aspiration on the syringe. After successful venipuncture with the finder needle, the large-bore needle is introduced in the identical plane.
- After cannulation, the guide wire is inserted through the large needle. Depth of insertion is limited to 15 to 20 cm to avoid arrhythmias.
- The central venous catheter is then threaded over the guide wire after using a scalpel to make a larger skin incision if needed and a dilator to dilate the subcutaneous tract.
- The guide wire is removed; the catheter is fixed with suture material and covered with sterile gauze.

Figure 4.5A shows various equipments required for CVC. **Figures 4.5A to D** show various steps of CVC.

Complications

The catheter should never be inserted through infected skin. Often there is significant risk of complications with this procedure, as follows:
- Hematoma formation
- Arrhythmias

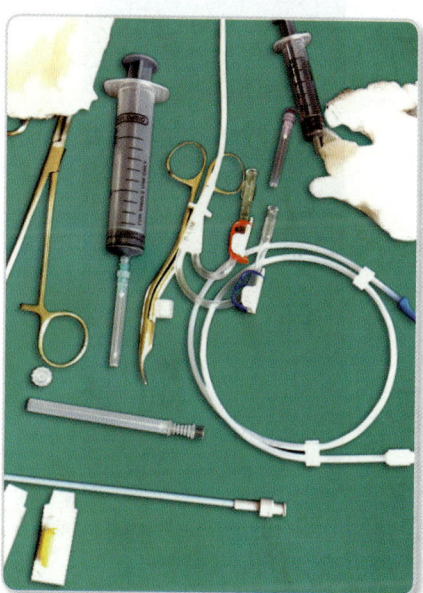

Figure 4.5A: Equipments required for central venous catheterization (*Courtesy:* Dr SY Hanjagi, Physician, Bijapur)

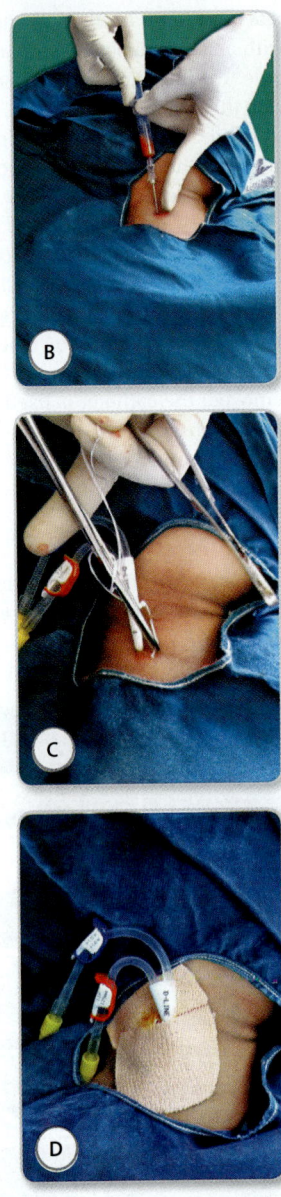

Figures 4.5B to D: Various steps of central venous catheterization
(*Courtesy:* Dr SY Hanjagi, Physician, Bijapur)

- Pneumothorax/hemothorax/hydrothorax
- Cardiac tamponade
- Air embolism
- Infection.

Arterial Catheterization

Indwelling arterial catheters allow performance of a number of important functions with relative safety and reliability.

Cannulation Sites

- Radial artery
- Dorsalis pedis artery
- Brachial artery
- Femoral artery
- Axillary artery.

Indications

- Hemodynamic monitoring.
- Frequent arterial blood gas sampling (>2 measurements/day).
- Arterial administration of drugs, such as thrombolytics.

Procedure

Radial Artery Cannulation

Modified Allen test is sometimes used to assess the extent of collateral flow through the ulnar artery. To perform this test, the examiner compresses both radial and ulnar arteries at wrist of one side and asks the patient to clench and unclench the fist repeatedly until pallor of the palm is observed. One artery is then released, and the time of appearance of erythema of the palm is noted. The procedure is repeated with the other artery.

The procedure for percutaneous insertion has been described below:

- The hand is placed in 30° to 60° of dorsiflexion. The volar aspect of the wrist is prepared and draped using the sterile technique and lidocaine is infiltrated through a 25 gauge needle.
- A 20 gauge, teflon 1.5" to 2" catheter-over-needle apparatus is used for the puncture. Insertion is made at 30° to 60° angle to the skin approximately 3 cm proximal to the distal wrist crease.
- The needle and cannula are advanced until arterial blood return is noted in the hub. A small amount of further advancement is necessary for the cannula to enter the artery as well.
- With this accomplished, needle and cannula are brought flat to the skin and the cannula is advanced to its hub with a firm, steady rotatory motion.
- Correct positioning is confirmed by pulsatile blood return on removal of the needle.

- The cannula is then secured firmly and attached to the transducer tubing. Antibiotic ointment is applied and the site is bandaged.

Complications
- Pain and swelling at the site.
- Thrombosis or embolism, leading to limb ischemia.
- Hemorrhage and hematoma formation.
- Infection.

AIRWAY ACCESS/MAINTENANCE

Introduction

Maintaining a patent airway is the first principle of resuscitation and life support. It is an essential skill for those caring for anesthetized or critically ill patients. Maintenance of upper airway patency is of paramount importance to prevent its obstruction and hypoxia. Airway management consists of techniques which clear the obstructed airway or bypass the obstruction, assist or replace spontaneous ventilation, permit tracheal suctioning and protect the lungs from soiling. Clinicians working in a hospital setting (respiratory care, nursing, intensive care, and emergency room physicians) must be competent in the basic essentials of airway care.

Opening of Airway

Functional suction apparatus is a must to handle the situation. However, effective manual maneuver will be additive to restore the proper airway.

Principles: When normal muscular control of the lower jaw and tongue is lost, the tongue may fall back against the posterior pharynx and obstruct the airway. Hence, manual maneuvers may be helpful.

Procedure

The Triple Airway Maneuver

It is the combination of head tilt, jaw thrust and opening of the mouth, and is the most reliable manual method to establish airway patency. When airway maneuvers are inadequate to establish airway patency, airway aids such as an 'oral or nasopharyngeal airways' should be used. If these maneuvers do not help, then definitive measures like tracheal intubation or tracheostomy should be done.

Head tilt: This is the simplest airway maneuver. The head is tilted back by placing one hand on the forehead and pushing down on the forehead. This approach should not be used in patients with a cervical spine injury or extensive cerebrovascular disease.

Chin lift: Fingers of the other hand are placed under the bony portion of the chin and the mandible is lifted upwards.

Procedures and Techniques in Dermatological Emergencies

Jaw thrust: This maneuver displaces the jaw forward by applying anterior pressure on the angle of the mandible. This procedure can be done in patients with suspected spinal injury.

Application of triple maneuver is the most effective and simple method for opening up of obstructed upper airway. Opening of airways by triple maneuver has been displayed in **Figures 4.6A and B and 4.7A and B.**

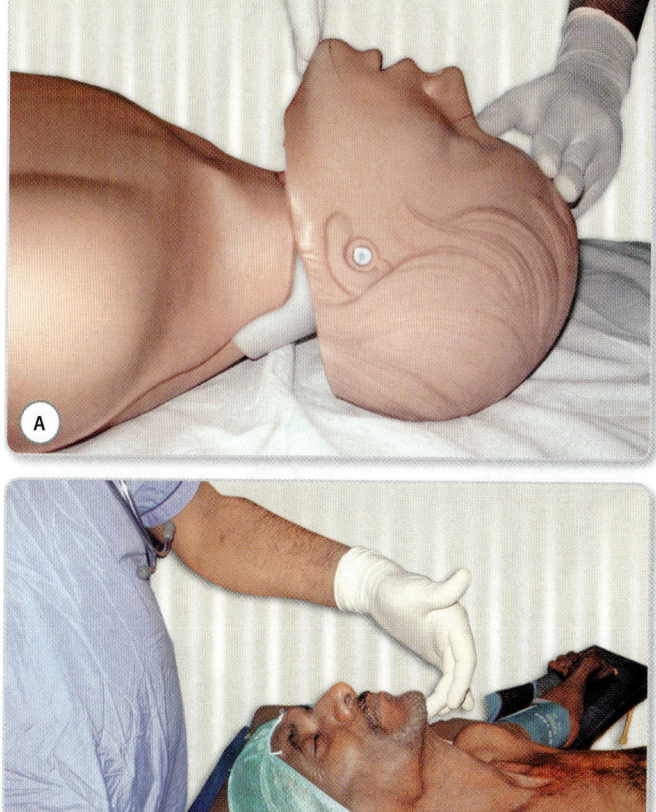

Figures 4.6A and B: Triple maneuver for opening of airways; head tilt and chin lift (A), chin lift (B)

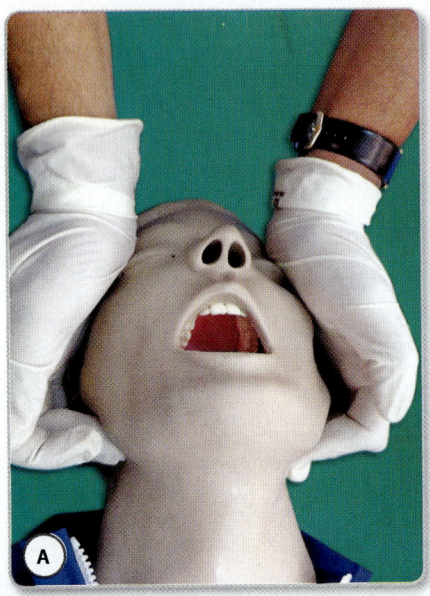

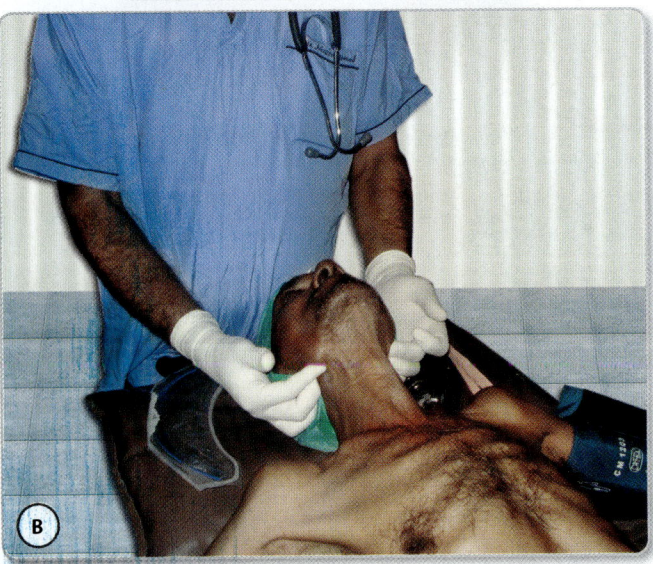

Figures 4.7A and B: Triple maneuver for opening of airways; jaw thrust *(Figure 4.7A, Courtesy:* Dr Vijay Katti, Anesthetist, Bijapur)

Monitoring and Care

The above described method is an emergency maneuver and needs to be replaced by definitive methods of maintaining the airways at the earliest.

Endotracheal Intubation

Endotracheal intubation is best achieved by intubation of the trachea with endotracheal tube. In case of difficult airway, supra glottic devices like 'laryngeal mask airway', 'combitube', etc. are used to control airway.

Indications

In critically ill patient, in semiconscious or unconscious state, vomitus or secretions may potentially obstruct the airway.
- Cardiac arrest of any etiology
- Unconscious patient
- Loss of airway patency or total airway obstruction as in,
  - Anaphylaxis
  - Angioedema involving laryngeal mucosa
  - Severe type 2 reaction in leprosy causing laryngeal edema and obstruction.

Equipment

Following is the list of equipments to be kept ready before starting the procedure; basic instruments necessary for endotracheal intubation has been displayed in **Figure 4.8**.
- A source of oxygen, face masks of different sizes, a bag-mask ventilation device and suction apparatus.
- Oral and nasopharyngeal airways.
- Laryngoscope blades and handle. Two basic types of laryngoscope blades are available: the curved blade (Macintosh) and the straight

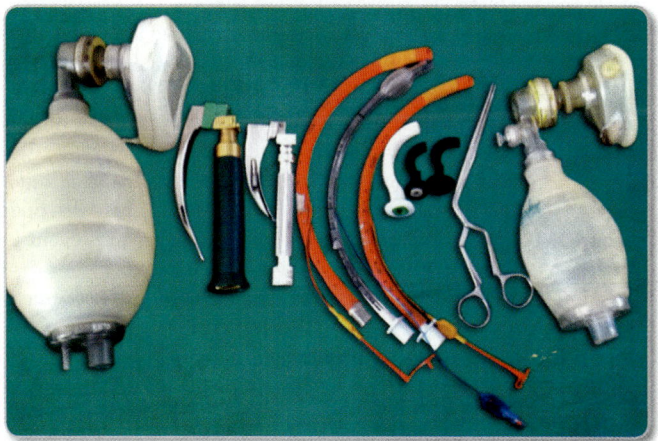

Figure 4.8: Equipments necessary for endotracheal intubation (from left to right: AMBU adult, laryngoscope adult and pediatric, endotracheal tubes [red rubber and portex], Guedal's oropharyngeal airway [adult and pediatric], Macgill's forceps, AMBU pediatrics) *(Courtesy:* Prof DG Talikoti, Anesthetist, Bijapur)

blade (Miller). The Miller blade is more useful in patients who have a cephalad and anterior laryngeal inlet.
- Various sizes of endotracheal tubes with stylets. The selection of proper tube diameter is very important. Endotracheal tube size 7.0 to 8.0 mm internal diameter is commonly used for adult women, while size 8.0 to 9.0 mm internal diameter tubes are used for adult men.
- A device to detect end-tidal carbon dioxide: colorimetric detector or capnograph.
- The required size of the endotracheal tubes used in children may be based on the formula:

$$\text{Endotracheal tube size (mm)} = [16 + \text{age (year)}]/4.$$

- Laryngeal mask airways (LMA) can be used to provide a temporary airway until a more definite airway can be achieved. The LMA is contraindicated in patients at risk of aspiration due to full stomach.

Conventional Orotracheal Intubation

Successful orotracheal intubation requires alignment of oral, pharyngeal, and laryngeal axes. The optimal position is the 'sniffing position'; the head is extended at atlanto-occipital joint and the neck is flexed.
- The laryngoscope handle is held in the left hand while the patient's mouth is opened as wide as possible. The laryngoscope blade is inserted into the right side of the mouth, the tongue is swept to the left and the blade is advanced forward towards the base of the tongue (**Figures 4.9A and B**). Lips are cleared if they are caught between the blade and the teeth.
- The curved blade is advanced into the vallecula and upward force at a 45° angle is used to raise the epiglottis. The straight blade is advanced and the tip of the blade is positioned beneath the epiglottis and upward force is applied in the same manner as with the curved blade. The blade should not be rotated back onto the teeth.
- Once the glottic opening is visualized, the endotracheal tube is advanced through the vocal cords until the cuff just disappears (**Figure 4.10A**). The cuff is inflated with enough air to prevent leak during positive-pressure ventilation (**Figure 4.10B**).
- Location of the tube in the trachea is confirmed. Signs of tracheal intubation consist of:
  - Presence of CO_2 in the exhaled breath,
  - Breath sounds over the chest,
  - Lack of breath sounds over the stomach,
  - Lack of gastric distention and
  - Presence of respiratory gas moisture in the endotracheal tube.
- Insertion of the tube to 23 cm at the incisors in males, and 21 cm in females generally provides optimal endotracheal tube position.

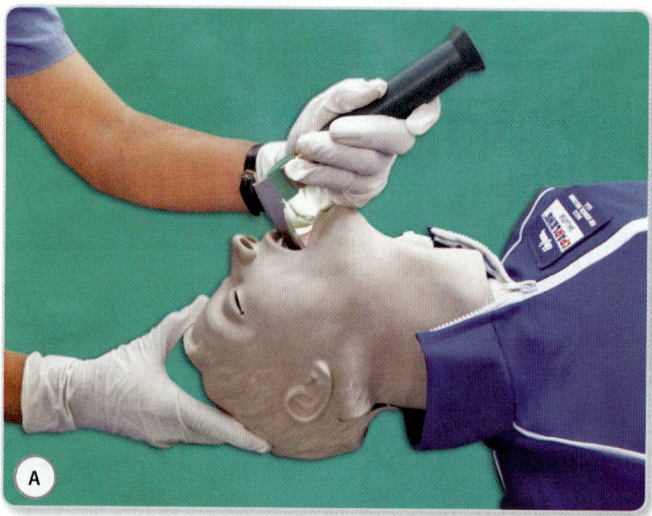

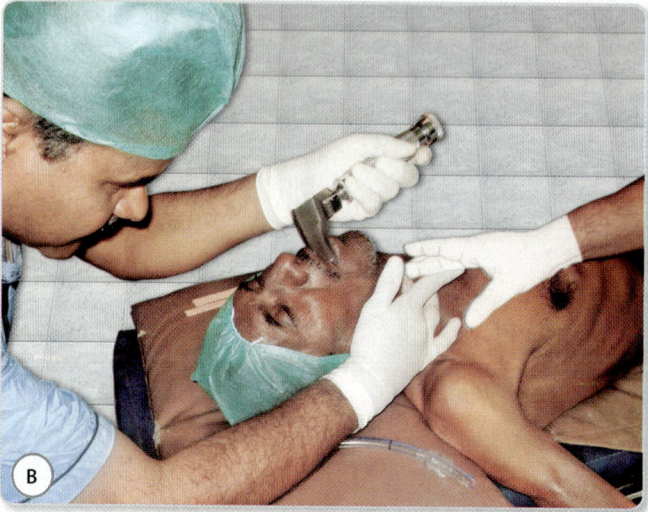

Figures 4.9A and B: Laryngoscope insertion; note the 'sniffing position' of the head
(Figure 4.9A, Courtesy: Dr Vijay Kumar TK, Anesthetist, Bijapur)

- In the unconscious patient who is considered to have a full stomach, laryngoscopy should be performed with cricoid pressure (*Sellick's maneuver*). Cricoid pressure should be applied by using the thumb and forefinger together to push downward on the cricoid cartilage. This maneuver can prevent passive regurgitation of stomach contents into the trachea during intubation.

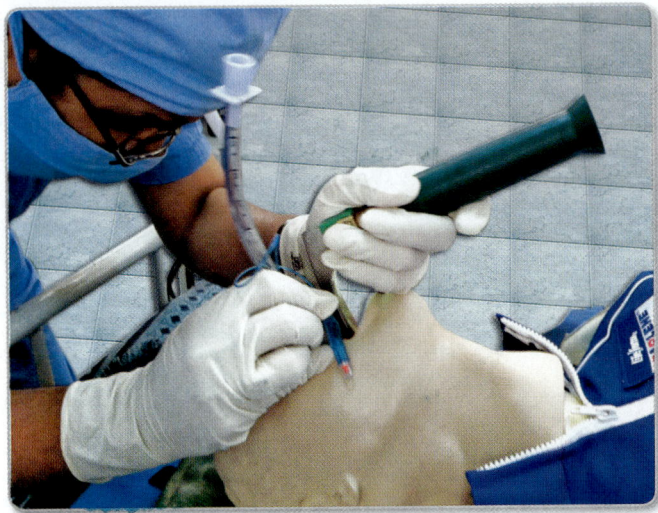

Figure 4.10A: Insertion of the endotracheal tube *(Courtesy:* Dr Vijay Katti, Anesthetist, Bijapur)

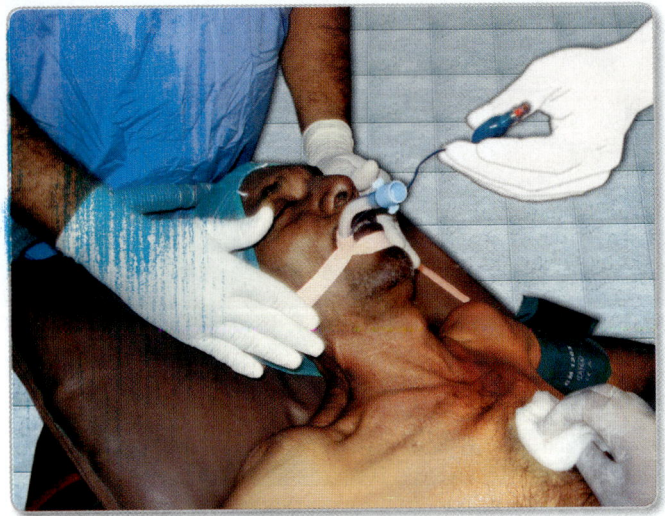

Figure 4.10B: Endotracheal tube in fixed position

Complications

Complications encountered during intubation and after extubation has been presented in **Table 4.1.**

Table 4.1: Complications arising due to endotracheal intubation

During intubation	After extubation
Laryngospasm	Laryngospasm
Laceration	Sore throat
Bruising of lips or tongue	Hoarseness
Damage to teeth	Stridor
Aspiration	Glottic or subglottic edema
Endobronchial or esophageal intubation	Tracheal stenosis
	Tracheomalacia
Perforation of oropharynx, trachea or esophagus	Tracheal mucosal ulceration
Epistaxis	

Nasotracheal Intubation

- The nasal approach generally provides the easier route for intubation.
- Topical vasoconstrictors such as phenylephrine or cocaine (4%) should be applied to the nares to minimize nasal bleeding.
- A well-lubricated, warmed tube with the cuff fully deflated should be inserted via either prepared nostril. Once the tube is beyond the nasopharynx, both blind and direct laryngoscopy techniques can be used to accomplish nasotracheal intubation.
- Nasotracheal intubation is contraindicated in basilar skull fractures, coagulopathies and intranasal abnormalities.

NASOGASTRIC ACCESS

Indications

Insertion of a nasogastric tube ensures access to the stomach and its contents. This serves following purpose:

- Drainage of gastric contents
- Decompression of the stomach
- Collection of specimen of the gastric contents
- Introduce a passage into the gastrointestinal tract for feeding.

Nasogastric intubation is helpful in patients admitted in DICU primarily for:

- Enteral feeding in patients with Stevens-Johnson syndrome-toxic epidermal necrolysis, immunobullous disorders/other critically ill patients
- For administering oral medications
- In treating gastric immobility and paralytic ileus
- For drainage of gastric contents
- For assessment of gastrointestinal bleeding.

Equipment

- Nasogastric/orogastric tube
- Syringe (60 ml) for tube tip irrigation
- Water-soluble lubricant, preferably 2% lignocaine jelly
- Adhesive tape
- Low powered suction device OR drainage bag
- Stethoscope
- Cup of water (if necessary)/ice chips
- Emesis basin
- pH indicator strips.

Basic equipments necessary for nasogastric tube insertion has been displayed in **Figure 4.11**.

Procedures of Nasogastric Tube Insertion

- Gloves should be worn.
- If patient is conscious the procedure is explained by showing the tube.
- If possible, the patient is made to sit upright for optimal neck/stomach alignment.
- Nostrils are examined for deformity/obstructions to determine better side for insertion.
- Tube is measured from bridge of the nose to earlobe, then to the point halfway between the end of the sternum and the umbilicus.
- Measured lengths are marked with a marker or the distance is noted.
- Using lubricant (preferably 2% lignocaine), 2-4" of the tube is lubricated. This procedure is very uncomfortable for many patients, so a squirt of lignocaine jelly in the nostril, and a spray of lignocaine to the back of the throat will help to alleviate the discomfort.

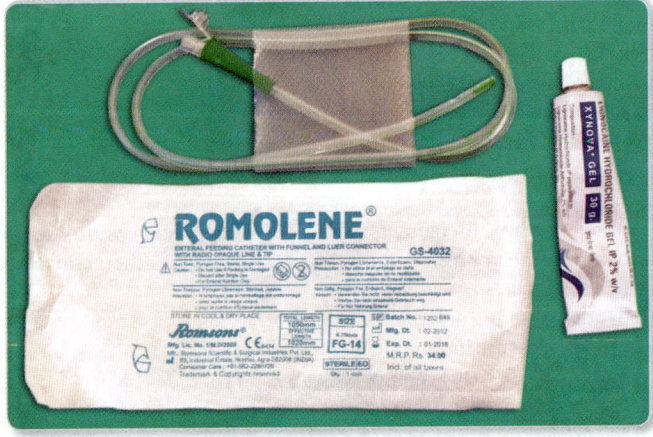

Figure 4.11: Equipments necessary for nasogastric tube insertion (Ryle's tube, lignocaine jelly) *(Courtesy:* Prof DG Talikoti, Anesthetist, Bijapur)

- The tube is passed through either of the nares posteriorly, past the pharynx into the esophagus and then to the stomach. (**Figure 4.12**).

The patient is instructed to make swallowing movement (ice chips/water may be offered to facilitate the process) and the tube is advanced as the patient does so. Swallowing of small sips of water may enhance passage of tube into esophagus.

If resistance is met, the tube is rotated slowly with downward advancement without extra force. The tube is withdrawn immediately:

- If there is change in patient's respiratory status,
- If the patient begins to cough or cyanosed
- If the tube coils inside the mouth.
- The tube is advanced until the mark is reached.
- Correct positioning of the tube is checked by attaching syringe to its free end and aspirating sample of gastric contents. Injection of air bolus is not recommended. The best practice is to test the pH of the aspirated contents (<6) to ensure that it is acidic. An x-ray may be taken to verify placement of the tube before instilling any feeding/medication or if there is any doubt about the position of the tube.
- The tube is secured with tape or commercially available tube holder.
- If meant for suction, the syringe is removed from the free end of the tube and connected to the suction machine. The machine is set for the type of suction and pressure as prescribed.
- Following are documented:
  - The reason for the tube insertion
  - Type and size of the tube

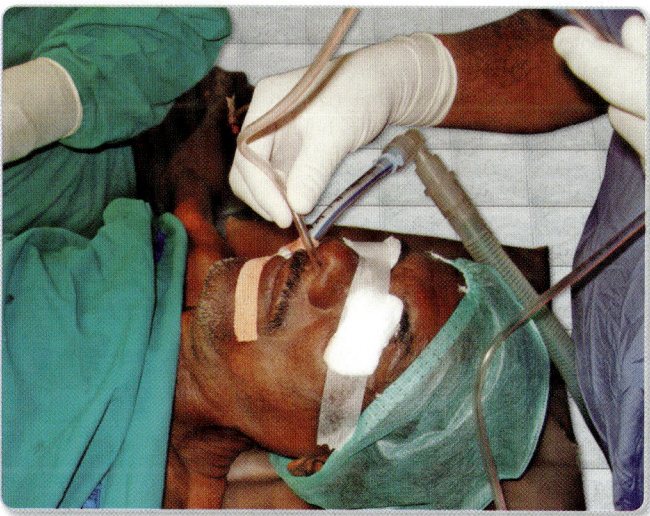

Figure 4.12: Nasogastric tube insertion

- Nature and amount of aspirate
- The type of suction and pressure setting if meant for suction
- The nature and amount of drainage.

Precaution

In patients with Stevens-Johnson syndrome/toxic epidermal necrolysis and immunobullous disorders extra care must be taken to insert the tube very gently as the oropharyngeal and esophageal mucosa is already friable and very painful.

Complications

The main complications of nasogastric intubation include aspiration and tissue trauma/perforation in presence of friable mucous membrane. Insertion of the tube may induce gagging or vomiting, therefore suction apparatus should always be ready to use in such situation.

TRANSURETHRAL CATHETERIZATION

Insertion of a urinary catheter is an essential skill in medicine, which must be adopted by all health care professionals. Catheters are sized in units termed 'French', where one French (FR) equals to 1/3rd of one mm. Catheters vary from 12 (small) FR to 48 (large) FR in size (3–16 mm). These also come in different varieties including ones without a bladder balloon, and the ones with different sized balloons. The capacity of the balloon when inflated with water, must be checked beforehand.

Indications

In patients with acute skin failure due to toxic epidermal necrolysis, immunobullous diseases, erythroderma, etc. where they are absolutely bedridden, transurethral catheterization or condom drainage is an absolute necessity. Moreover, it is helpful to maintain the output chart accurately.

Equipment

- Sterile gloves
- Sterile drapes
- Cleansing solution
- Cotton swabs
- Forceps
- Sterile water (usually 10 cc)
- Foley catheter (usually 16–18 French)
- Syringe (usually 10 cc)
- Lubricant (water-based jelly or lignocaine jelly)
- Collection bag and tubing.

Procedure

- In conscious patients, the procedure is explained.
- Patient is assisted into supine position with legs spread and feet together.
- Catheterization set and catheter is opened.
- Sterile field is prepared, sterile gloves worn.
- Catheter balloon is checked for patency and size.
- The distal portion (2–5 cm) of the catheter is generously coated with lubricant.
- Sterile drape is applied.
- If female, labia are separated using nondominant hand. If male, the penis is held with the nondominant hand. Hand position is maintained until preparing to inflate the balloon.
- Using dominant hand to hold forceps, periurethral mucosa is cleaned with cleansing solution. Cleansing is done anterior to posterior, inner to outer, one swipe per swab, and swab is discarded away from the sterile field.
- Catheter is taken with gloved dominant hand. End of catheter is held loosely coiled in palm of the dominant hand.
- In male, the penis is lifted to a position perpendicular to patient's body and light upward traction is applied (with nondominant hand).
- Urinary meatus is identified and the catheter is gently inserted up to 1 to 2" beyond where urine is noted (**Figure 4.13A**).
- Balloon is inflated using correct amount of sterile liquid (usually 10 cc) (**Figure 4.13B**).
- The catheter is gently pulled until inflated balloon is snug against the bladder neck.
- Catheter is connected to urobag.
- Catheter is secured to abdomen or thigh, without tension on tubing.
- Drainage bag is placed below the level of bladder.
- Catheter function and drained urine (amount, color, other characters) is evaluated.
- Gloves removed and the equipments disposed appropriately followed by handwash.
- Size of catheter inserted, amount of water in balloon and assessment of urine is documented.

Complications

The most common short-term complication of urinary catheterization is inability to insert the catheter, causing tissue trauma during the insertion. The major complication is infection. After 48 hours of catheterization, most catheters are colonized with bacteria, thus leading to possible bacteriuria and its complications. Catheters can also cause renal inflammation, nephro-cystolithiasis, and pyelonephritis if left in for prolonged period.

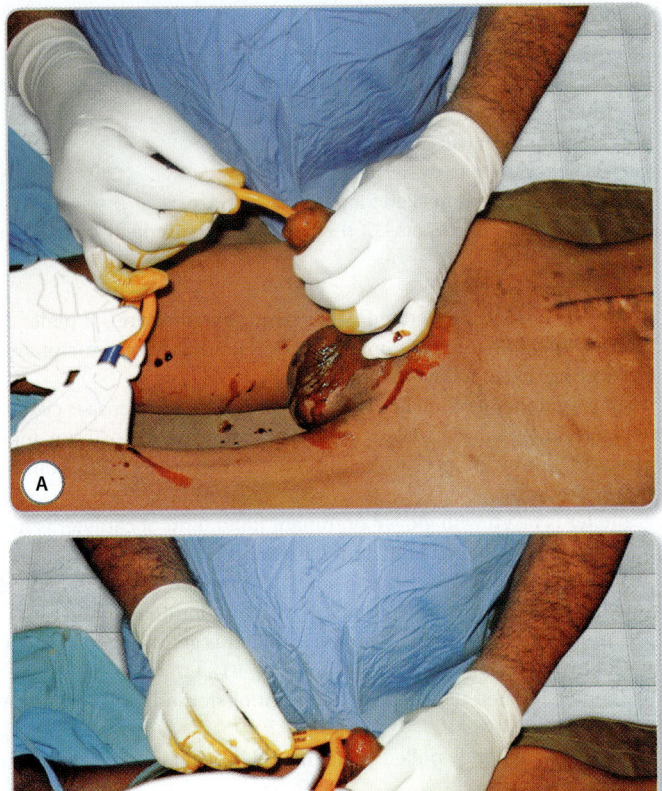

Figures 4.13A and B: Transurethral catheterization and inflation of the balloon

The alternatives to urethral catheterization include suprapubic catheterization and external condom catheters for longer durations.

Condom Drainage

This may be practiced in nonambulant conscious and unconscious male patients for urinary drainage (**Figure 4.13C**). A latex condom is unrolled on penis, fixed with adhesive tape and its tip is pierced with the urobag

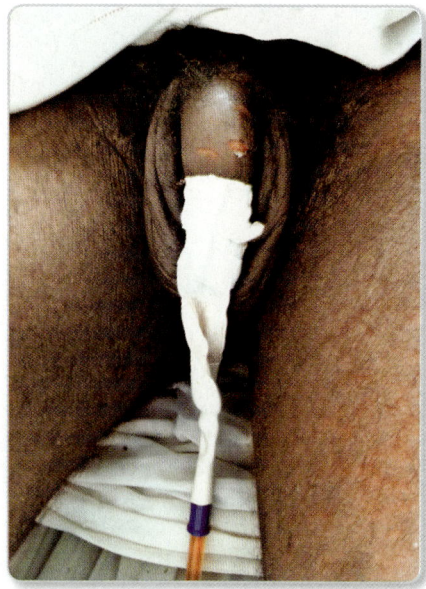

Figure 4.13C: Condom drainage in a patient with drug hypersensitivity syndrome

tubing (fixed with adhesive tape). The risk of urinary tract infection due to catheterization may be avoided by this method.

In neonates and pediatric patients neonatal and pediatric 'urine collectors' may be used for collection of urine (**Figures 4.13D and E**).

CARDIOPULMONARY RESUSCITATION

A. Basic life support
B. Advanced cardiac life support

Advanced life support requires adequate skill and efficiency. Here 'basic life support' which may be performed by a dermatologist in ICU (following adequate training) has been discussed.

Basic Life Support

Basic life support (BLS) is the foundation for saving lives following cardiac or respiratory arrest. Fundamental aspects of BLS include immediate **recognition** of sudden cardiac arrest (SCA) and **activation** of the emergency response system, early **cardiopulmonary resuscitation** (CPR), and rapid **defibrillation** with an automated external defibrillator (AED). The principles of basic life support (BLS) have been represented diagrammatically in **Figure 4.14**.

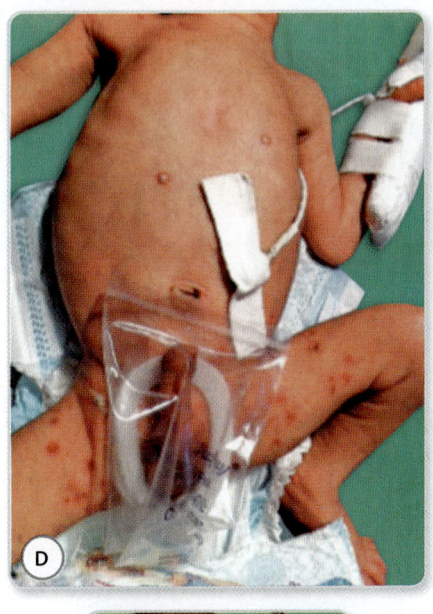

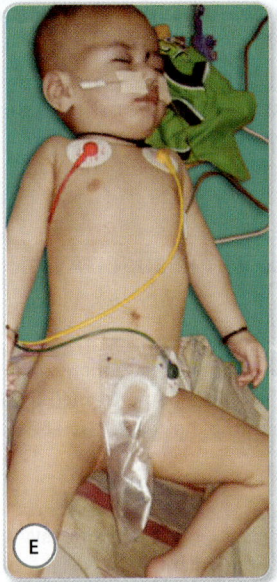

Figures 4.13D and E: Neonatal and pediatric urine collectors

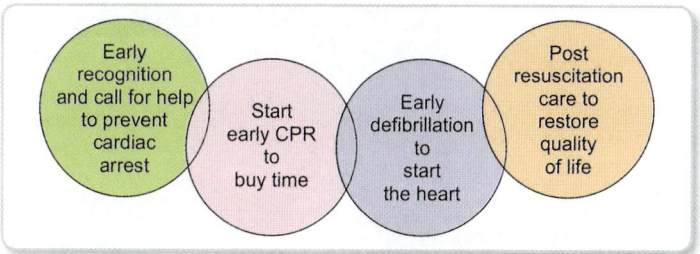

Figure 4.14: Chain of survival

CPR is a basic, life saving technique for sudden cardiac or respiratory arrest and it involves a combination of rescue breathing and chest compressions. CPR relies on three basic rescue skills:

A Airway
B Breathing
C Circulation

The purpose of CPR is to keep the oxygenated blood supply intact to the person's brain and heart until qualified medical help arrives. Any trained individual can perform CPR. Timely intervention may make a difference in patient survival. The sequence of life saving procedures to be performed **(Figures 4.15, 4.16A and B and 4.17)** in a patient with sudden cardiac and/or pulmonary arrest has been presented in **Table 4.2**.

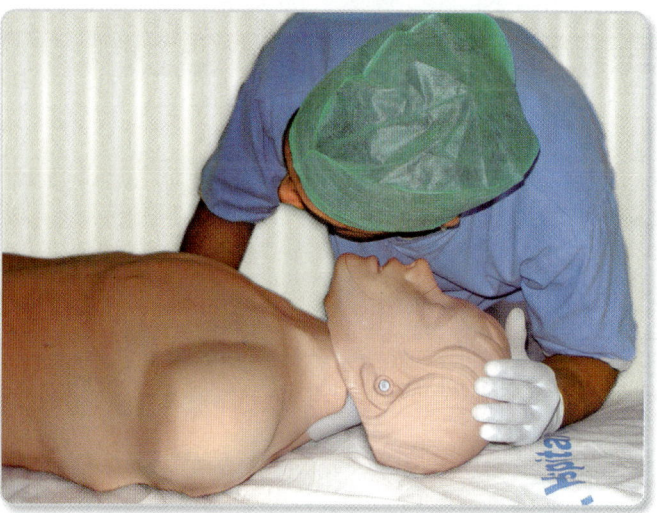

Figure 4.15: Look, listen and feel for breathing

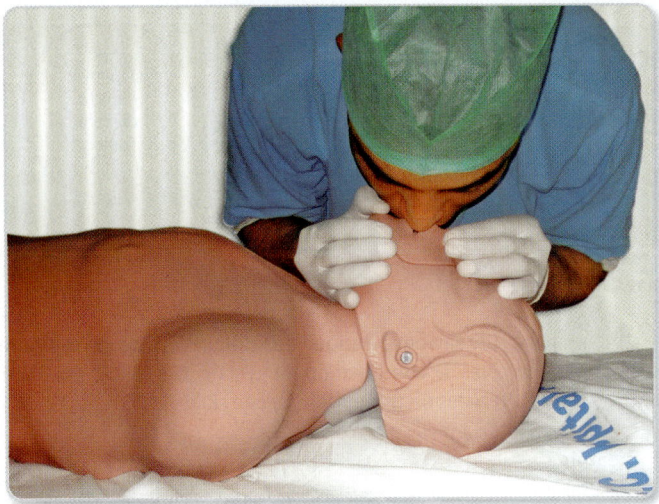

Figure 4.16A: Rescue mouth to mouth breath

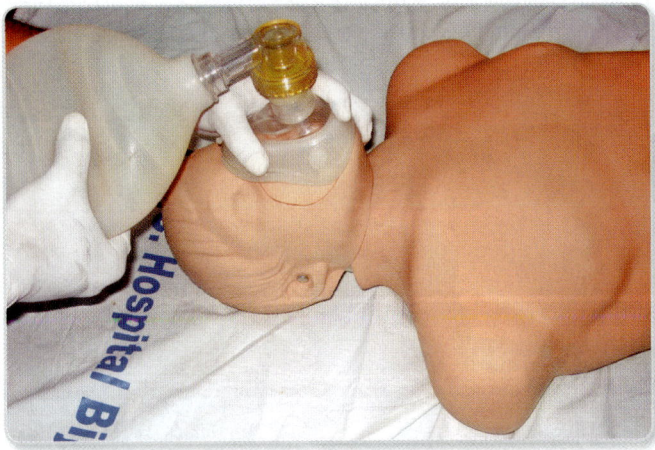

Figure 4.16B: Rescue breath with AMBU bag

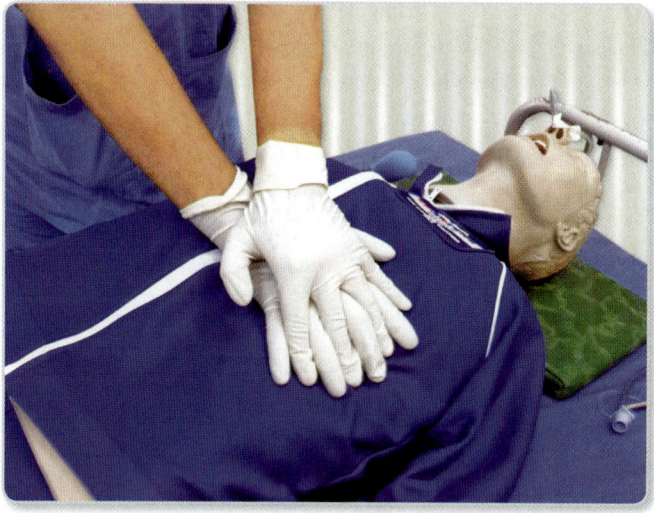

Figure 4.17: Chest compressions *(Courtesy:* Dr Vijay Katti, Anesthetist, Bijapur)

Table 4.2: Sequence of life saving procedures to be performed in a patient with sudden cardiac and or pulmonary arrest in DICU

Sequence	Critical actions
1. Check response	If unresponsive act quickly!
2. Establish an open airway **(A)**	Head tilt, chin lift + jaw thrust
3. Check breathing **(B)**	a. Look for chest movement, listen for breath sounds and feel for exhaled breath (**Figure 4.15**) b. Do not confuse agonal breathing with normal breathing
Give effective **Two rescue breaths** (Tidal volume 500–600 ml)	• Pinch the nose (**Figure 4.16**) • Take a normal breath • Place lips over mouth or use AMBU bag (**Figures 4.16A and B**) • Blow until the chest rises • Take about 1 second • Allow chest to fall

Contd...

Contd...

Sequence	Critical actions
4. Check for circulation (**C**)	Determine pulselessness by feeling for carotid or femoral pulse

a. Give effective **Thirty chest compressions**	• Place the heel of one hand in the center of the chest
	• Place other hand on top
	• Interlock fingers
	• Compress the chest (**Figure 4.17**)
	  – Rate 100/min
	  – Depth 4–5 cm
	  – Equal compression: relaxation
	• When possible change CPR operator every 2 minutes
	Provide Compression/Ventilation ratio of **30:2 per cycle**
	Reassess circulation after completion of **5 cycles of CPR (2 min)**

5. Early defibrillation	Use automated external defibrillator (AED)

6. Continue CPR	Continue **30 chest compressions** and **2 rescue breaths until**
	  – Qualified help arrives and takes over
	  – The patient starts breathing normally
	  – Rescuer becomes exhausted

In conclusion, though CPR is the domain of anesthetists in routine medical practice, during an emergency situation an anesthetist may not be available on the spot. Hence, each and every member of the DICU team must be conversant with minimum basic life saving techniques so that a patient's life can be saved at any point of time. At the time of setting up a DICU, a prior hands-on training course for all the members of DICU team should be made mandatory.

ACKNOWLEDGEMENT

I hereby acknowledge the help of Dr Satish S Kallatti, postgraduate student in the department of anesthesiology, for taking the clinical photographs.

SUGGESTED FURTHER READING

1. Berg RA, Hemphill R, Abella BS, Aufderheide TP, Cave DM, Hazinski MF, et al. Adult basic life support:2010. American Heart Association Guidelines for CPR and emergency cardiovascular care. Circulation 2010;122:685–705.

2. Marino PL. Vascular access. In: Marino PL, Sutin KM, editors. The ICU book, 3rd edition. Pennsylvania:Lippincott Williams & Wilkins; 2006.p-121-43.
3. Orebaugh SL. Direct laryngoscopy. In: Orebaugh SL, editor. In: Atlas airway management: techniques and tools, 1st edition. Pennsylvania: Lippincott Williams & Wilkins; 2007.p-14-22.
4. Webster PA, Salassi-Scotter MR. Peripheral vascular access. In: Dieckmann RA, Fiser DH, Selbst SM, editors. Illustrated textbook of pediatric emergency and critical care procedures. St. Louis, Missouri: Mosby-Year Book; 1997.p-187-202.
5. Young KK, Oh TE. Airway management. In: Oh TE, editor. Intensive care Manual, 4th edition. Edinburgh: Butterworth Heinmann; 1998.p-217-27.

chapter 5

Diagnostic Procedures in Critical Care Set Up

BV Peerapur

- Blood culture
- Pus sample collection
- Specimen collection from skin
- Specimen collection from throat and mouth
- Specimen collection from rectum
- Bedside estimation of bleeding time and clotting time

INTRODUCTION

While a patient is under treatment in a dermatological intensive care unit (DICU), it is necessary to investigate the patient for various infections. The cause of infection in a patient admitted in DICU may be as follows:

- The infection may be the patient's primary illness necessitating admission, as in meningococcemia, necrotizing fasciitis, staphylococcal scalded skin syndrome.
- Underlying infection might have precipitated the dermatological emergency, necessitating admission, as in acute infectious purpura fulminans.
- Associated infection (present during admission or nosocomial), which might have worsened patient's primary illness, as in;
  - Erythroderma of any etiology.
  - Disorders resulting in large areas of skin erosion, e.g. pemphigus, epidermolysis bullosa, Stevens-Johnson syndrome (SJS), toxic epidermal necrolysis (TEN).

Nosocomial infections may be cutaneous and systemic. The source of cutaneous nosocomial infection may be contaminated hospital environment and carrier health care workers. Important routes for acquiring systemic nosocomial infection are intravenous cannula, and urinary catheter.

In the following section some of the procedures have been described, which are necessary to detect or rule out infection in patients admitted in DICU.

BLOOD CULTURE

Blood culture for presence of bacteria and fungi is considered as one of the most important investigations to be performed in patients receiving treatment in a critical care set up.

Indications for Blood Culture

Blood culture should be performed on any patient in whom there is a suspicion of septicemia or invasive fungimia.

Following are the indications of blood culture in a patient admitted in DICU:
1. Evident cutaneous infection (pus collection) with marked systemic features and poor response to antibiotic.
2. Patients with erythroderma/acute skin failure in whom sepsis is suspected because of;
   - persistent fever,
   - sudden hypothermia in a febrile patient,
   - persistent tachycardia,
   - persistent hypotension,
   - sudden anuria.
3. Suspected disseminated gonococcal infection.
4. Suspected meningococcemia.
5. Suspected candidemia or disseminated cryptococcosis in patients for whom routine cultures have not detected *Candida* species or *Cryptococcus neoformans*, respectively.
6. Suspected invasive infection by *Malassezia furfur* originating in IV cannula, in patients receiving intravenous lipid transfusion.

Principles of Sample Collection for Blood Culture

- Blood should not be collected from indwelling arterial or venous lines unless an infected intravenous line is suspected. If blood is drawn for culture from an indwelling line, a second specimen should be obtained from a peripheral site.
- Two or more blood samples should be collected using sterile technique at separate sites, before starting antibiotics. Except in very unusual cases, no more than 3 sets of blood cultures should be collected within 24 hours period. If all the 3 samples are negative after 24 hours and sepsis is still suspected, more samples may be collected.
- A larger number of blood culture samples may have to be collected from persons already receiving antimicrobials. If patient's clinical condition permits, stopping antibiotics and repeat blood culture after 48 hours is preferred.
- In adults, ideally a minimum of 10 ml of blood, depending on the blood culture system used, should be inoculated into a culture

bottle. Adequate volume of blood improves detection of pathogenic organisms and reduces time for detection.
- Arterial blood sample provides no advantage over venous samples.

Technique of Sample Collection for Blood Culture

- A proper peripheral venous site is chosen.
- Antiseptic dressing is done to the area and it is allowed to dry.
- Blood sample is collected using sterile disposable syringe and needle with gloved hands.
- The needle is removed from the syringe and the blood is collected into sterile blood culture bottle (both aerobic and anaerobic). The collected specimen is sent to laboratory immediately.

PUS SAMPLE COLLECTION

Presence of pus in skin lesions is suggestive of active infection. Gram stain and culture sensitivity test of pus helps in detecting the causative organism and making therapeutic decision.

Following are the principles of pus sample collection from a patient:

- Sterile gloves are worn and sterile culture tube with cotton-tipped swab stick is kept ready.
- Preferably sample is collected before starting any topical and systemic antibiotic, during the acute stage of the disease. Pus should never be collected from containers like drainage bag/bottle.
- Appropriate site for collection of pus is selected. It may be difficult in patients with widespread cutaneous involvement like Stevens-Johnson syndrome, toxic epidermal necrolysis, pemphigus and erythroderma, where frank pus may not be visible. In such situations, an oozy area of skin is preferably selected. In patients with staphylococcal scalded skin syndrome, sampling should be done from nasal vestibule or conjunctiva, as the organism is not present in skin lesions.
- The lesion or the area of skin is cleaned with normal saline swab. If a yet unruptured abscess is seen pus may be aspirated with a sterile, disposable syringe and needle and transferred to the culture tube. From other areas pus collection is done using the cotton-tipped swab stick, with due care to collect adequate quantity of sample. The swab is transferred to the culture tube immediately and sent to laboratory without delay with a requisition form carrying patient details.
- The sample is inoculated for both aerobic and anaerobic cultures.

SPECIMEN COLLECTION FROM SKIN

Skin sample is collected in patients with breach of skin surface continuity, as in erythroderma or SJS-TEN, in absence of visible focus of infection. These patients are susceptible to develop fatal septicemia and requires close monitoring of skin surface microflora. Following are the indications of sample collection from skin in patients with dermatological emergencies:

- In patients with septicemia without evidence of active focus of infection (cutaneous/systemic).
- In patients with erythroderma/SJS-TEN, pemphigus and epidermolysis bullosa, as part of routine patient monitoring microbiological specimen from skin is collected at regular intervals.
- In patients with staphylococcal scalded skin syndrome.

Following steps are followed while collecting specimen from skin:

- The area from where specimen is to be collected is cleaned with a wet gauze piece (without any antiseptic).
- Swab stick moistened with normal saline or sterile nutrient broth is taken for sample collection. It is rolled firmly over the area. If crusts and scabs are present, these are removed gently with the help of a sterile plain forceps and collected in a sterile test tube or capped bottle. The collected specimen is immediately sent to laboratory.

SPECIMEN COLLECTION FROM THROAT AND MOUTH

Throat and mouth swabs should preferably be collected by an experienced nurse or treating doctor. Indications for throat and mouth swab collection in patients admitted in DICU are as follows:

- Patients with severe oral erosions as in SJS-TEN and pemphigus, to rule out any superadded bacterial or fungal infection, which may impair the healing of the lesions.
- In patients admitted in DICU and concomitant septicemia, to rule out oropharyngeal focus of infection.
- In patients with suspected disseminated gonococcal infection, where pharynx may be a focus of infection.

Technique of Specimen Collection

- For 8 hours before specimen collection, the patient must not be treated with antibiotics or antiseptic mouthwashes (gargles).
- Using tongue depressor, inner aspect of mouth is examined with the help of a good light source. Evidence of inflammation, presence of any membrane, exudate or pus should be looked for.
- Specimen is collected from the affected area using a sterile cotton swab, taking care not to contaminate the swab with saliva, and it is returned to the sterile container.
- Within two hours of collection, the specimen must be sent to the laboratory.

SPECIMEN COLLECTION FROM RECTUM

Rectal specimen collection may be required in patients with suspected disseminated gonococcal infection, where gram stain and culture of urethral/cervical or pharyngeal specimens are inconclusive.

Sample should be taken from the mucosa of distal rectum. Sterile cotton-tipped/alginate swab stick (approx. 11" long) is used to collect specimens from rectum (exudate and mucus).

- In patients with anorectal symptoms, ideally the sample should be taken using anoscope to enhance the possibility of isolation of gonococci both by gram stain and culture.
- In patients without anorectal symptoms, the swab stick may be inserted blindly up to 2 to 3 cm into the rectum and the specimen is collected.

The swab stick must be rolled side to side to collect samples from the crypts. If fecal soiling occurs, the swab stick is discarded and fresh specimen collected.

Sensitivity of both the procedures of collection of specimens appears to be equal. Care should be taken to avoid unnecessary contamination of the specimen with bacteria from the anal skin.

Selective media used to culture *N. gonorrhoeae* is modified Thayer-Martin media which normally contains vancomycin and colistin to inhibit growth of other bacteria. When rectal specimen is inoculated, trimethoprim is usually added to inhibit growth of *Proteus sp.* as the other antibacterials present in the media does not inhibit this organism.

BEDSIDE ESTIMATION OF BLEEDING TIME AND CLOTTING TIME

Estimation of bleeding time (BT) and clotting time (CT) at bedside are rapid methods to assess platelet function and integrity of intrinsic clotting system, respectively.

Estimation of Bleeding Time

Equipments required: Sphygmomanometer, micro lancet with disposable needles, stop watch, cotton swab and gloves. Following are the steps for estimation of BT:

- Sphygmomanometer cuff is wrapped around patient's arm and the mercury column is raised up to 40 mm Hg and maintained at that level during the period of the test.
- A prick (depth 2.5 mm and width 1 mm) is made on volar aspect of the same forearm, using the micro lancet.
- The stop watch is started as soon as blood starts oozing from the wound.

- Blood oozing from the wound is gently wiped off repeatedly (with gloved hand) using cotton swab till the bleeding stops and the stop watch is stopped at this point.
- The wound is occluded with a small dressing and adhesive tape.
- The time recorded in the stop watch from beginning to stoppage of bleeding is recorded as bleeding time.
- Normal bleeding time ranges from 2 to 7 minutes. An increase in BT should be confirmed by platelet count and/or functional assay of platelets.

Indications of estimation of BT in dermatological emergencies: Purpura fulminans, Kassabach-Merritt syndrome, meningococcemia (in presence of disseminated intravascular coagulation), Rickettsial spotted fever, dengue hemorrhagic fever and dengue shock syndrome, toxic shock syndrome (in presence of thrombocytopenia), etc.

Estimation of Clotting Time

Lee and White method of estimating CT has been described below.
Equipments required: Unsiliconized glass tube with external bore of 10 mm, disposable syringe with needle, stop watch, cotton swab soaked with spirit and gloves. Following steps are followed:

- The glass tubes are prewarmed at 37° C in a water bath.
- Blood (2–2.5 ml) is withdrawn from antecubital vein by single puncture using a disposable syringe and needle.
- The stop watch is started as soon as the blood enters the syringe.
- One ml blood is poured into the tube directly from the syringe after removal of the needle.
- The tube is kept at 37° C for 2 minutes and thereafter it is tilted every minute to see for flowing of blood within the tube. The process is continued till the tube can be tilted at more than 90° angle without spilling of blood and the stop watch is stopped at this point.
- The time interval recorded is the clotting time.
- Normal CT is 4 to 9 minutes. An increase in CT should be confirmed by coagulation profile. Sensitivity of estimation of CT is low as it is prolonged only in severe coagulation disorders.

Indications of estimation of CT in dermatological emergencies include:
Purpura fulminans, antiphospholipid antibody syndrome, Kassabach-Merritt syndrome, meningococcemia (in presence of disseminated intravascular coagulation), dengue hemorrhagic fever and dengue shock syndrome, toxic shock syndrome (in presence of disseminated intravascular coagulation), etc.

In conclusion, dermatologists should adopt the basic methods of bedside investigations and various techniques of sample collection for laboratory investigations as described above. In addition to bedside estimation of BT and CT, dermatologists should also be conversant with some other simple techniques like, detection of urinary protein and sugar, urine microscopy, examination of peripheral blood smear and measuring ESR. If these tests can be performed in the DICU, it may help in rapid decision making in a critically ill patient.

SUGGESTED FURTHER READING

1. Baron EJ, Peterson LR, Finegold SM. Selection, collection and transport of specimens for microbiological examination. In: Baron EJ, Peterson LR, Finegold SM, editors. Bailey & Scott's diagnostic microbiology, 9th edition. St Louis: Mosby; 1994.p-53-64.
2. Murray PR, Witebsky FG. The clinician and the microbiology laboratory. In:Mandell GL, Bennett JE, Dolin R, editors. Mandell, Douglas and Bennett's principles and practice of infectious diseases, 7th edition, vol-1. Philadelphia: Churchill Livingstone Elsevier; 2010.p-233-65.
3. Rausch M, Remley JG. General concepts in specimen collection and handling. In: Mahon CR, Manuselis G, editors. Textbook of diagnostic microbiology, 2nd edition. Philadelphia: W.B.Saunders Company; 2000. p-237-60.
4. Sinha SK. Disorders of haemostasis. In: Sanyal S, Bhattacharyya A, editors. Clinical pathology. A practical manual, 2nd edition. New Delhi: Elsevier; 2008.p-179-87.
5. Thomas PA. Collection and transport of specimens for microbiological examination. In: Ananthanarayan R, Paniker CKJ, editors. Ananthanarayan and Paniker's textbook of microbiology, 8th edition. Hyderabad: Universities Press; 2009.p-646-51.

chapter 6

Nursing Care in Dermatological Emergencies

Vineet Kaur

- Nursing care of the skin in non-dermatological critically ill patients
- Nursing care of the skin in dermatological emergencies

INTRODUCTION

The term 'emergency' is not usually associated with the skin. For dermatologists, acute skin failure is a relatively new concept, being described as recently as 1991 by Irvine and Ryan. For others in the field of medicine, it is a non-entity. In spite of being the largest and most visible organ of the body, it is seen as being associated with only chronic, self-limiting or recurrent conditions with negligible mortality potential. However, any health care professional, patient or caregiver who has ever encountered one of the conditions discussed in the subsequent sections, would agree that the challenge of caring for such skin is enormous. Since there are very few specialist centers geared to deal with dermatological emergencies in most parts of the world, there is very little literature available on this subject.

Acute skin failure is as much a medical emergency as any other organ failure since the skin performs the vital functions that control the overall hemostasis of the body. Being the first line of physical defense, a loss of this barrier function has huge implications for fluid regulation, temperature control, infection control, metabolism and nutrient balance. A study in UK has highlighted the fact that patients with skin conditions necessitating intensive care unit (ICU) admission have a higher mortality and longer average stay, providing further evidence for the importance of skin failure as a distinct entity. The eventual outcome of the patient in these situations is a result of the combined efforts of a team including dermatologists, intensivists and dedicated, trained nurses. Increasingly, the role of the critical skin care nurse is being highlighted in centers of excellence around the world.

Skin care nursing as a specialty is firmly established in some 'developed' parts of the world, is in its infancy in others and does not exist at all in yet others. Whilst there may be patients who have access to the most advanced nursing care in conditions of dermatological emergencies within specialized ICU earmarked for such patients, at the other extreme there may be some who do not have even the most basic facilities required to protect such skin. This poses a huge challenge in the transfer of knowledge between these vastly different situations. In the ideal world, one would wish for a uniformly good level of competence amongst health care professionals caring for the skin and the availability of resources. However, in the absence of such a luxury, every effort must be made to arrive at a bare minimum level of expertise in caring for patients with acute skin failure.

The guiding principles for care in these patients are universal. The aim is to understand the physiological changes that occur when the skin fails and work towards the correction. In order to ensure a successful outcome, the nurse needs to work in tandem with the medical team with utmost diligence. It is a good idea to have shorter working shifts for intensive care nurses based on the sheer intensity of the nursing process. A tired nurse can never contribute favorably to a better outcome.

The following discussion on skin care in the critically ill will be discussed in two sections:

- Skin care nursing in non-dermatological critically ill patients
- Nursing care of patients with dermatological emergencies.

SKIN CARE NURSING IN NON-DERMATOLOGICAL CRITICALLY ILL PATIENTS

Whenever a patient is admitted to an ICU for medical or surgical conditions, there are always issues linked to skin care nursing. Following facts call for special attention to these patients' skin:

- Such patients are largely bedridden.
- May have poor tissue perfusion as in low cardiac output states.
- Nutritionally and immunologically compromised.
- May have multiple infusion sites.
- May be intubated and/or catheterized.
- May have ostomies or surgical wounds.

An entity that is now gaining notice in patients admitted in ICU is perineal dermatitis. Fecal and urinary incontinence is the most common underlying cause for this condition. Studies have shown that up to a third of patients with fecal incontinence develop perineal dermatitis.

Age is a factor that influences skin breakdown. Extremes of age are the most vulnerable. In the elderly, the presence of underlying chronic diseases compounds the impact of an acute illness and hastens skin breakdown. In the pediatric age group, the commonest complication of the critically ill child's skin is pressure ulcers. Their incidence has been estimated to be up to 7% in acutely ill children. In infants and children, the commonest sites for these ulcers are the head and heels which are different from the adult and elderly population where sacral ulcers are the commonest.

Discussed below are some of the common conditions likely to be encountered in the critically ill patients and the care of the skin in such situations.

Pressure Ulcers

Pressure ulcers are one of the most underrated medical problems in critically ill patients. The lack of a risk assessment scale uniquely designed to determine the risk in these patients is an impediment to their prevention to a large extent. The fact that critically ill patients cannot reposition themselves and thus are totally dependent on nurses and care givers to move themselves, puts them at high risk for shearing injuries. In spite of advocates of glide sheets and patient transfer devices, there continues to be a significant incidence of pressure ulcers especially in the sacral areas. Many studies have shown that the risk of development of pressure ulcers is directly linked to the duration of hospital stay. The most physiologically unstable time for the patient is the first week in the ICU. Multiple life saving procedures and devices are being used to stabilize the patient and so there is much movement, pulling and shifting. Nurses in ICU have to be hyper-vigilant not only in terms of care of vitals but also regarding keen observation of the skin. During this period there should be very effective communication between all members of the health care team especially during change of shifts. The earliest signs of an impending pressure ulcer must be reported to the medical team and corrective steps instituted.

Nurses' role in prevention of pressure ulcer:
- A full skin assessment on admission of the patient and then follow-up at 12 hourly intervals or at the time of change.
- Recording of any sign of skin breakdown and communication to the member of nursing staff taking over the charge of next shift.
- Involvement with the medical team in planning a care protocol.
- Clear instructions on periodic repositioning.
- Exact description of reposition including any devices to off load pressure.
- Close monitoring of nutritional intake and coordination with nutritionist.
- Management of moisture from incontinence; incontinence pads, barrier creams.
- Use of skin sealants in 'at risk' areas of skin.
- Close check of skin under medical devices like intubation apparatus, oxygen delivery equipment, etc. to identify early onset of pressure ulcers from these devices.

A special mention of repositioning is necessary. Most pressure ulcers occur due to shearing stress on the skin during repositioning. Nurses in the ICU must take utmost care to avoid this by using transfer devices. They should be aware of potential areas of pressure, given the medical condition of the individual patient. Strict instructions on patient repositioning need to be given in cases of spinal instability. Often various life saving equipments can pose a great challenge to repositioning and nurses must be fully competent to handle these equipments, should they get disturbed during a position change. Frequent repositioning, 2 hourly ideally, is crucial. A 30° left lateral position is best for most ICU patients but there must be heel and shoulder support. Some patients might have to be nursed in a prone position.

One of the commonest complications seen in pediatric ICUs (PICU) is pressure ulcers. One study estimated the incidence to be up to >10%. Strategies associated with reducing their occurrence are largely similar to those in adults except that devices like egg craters and convoluted foam overlays are more commonly used in the PICU. The fact that due to differing body proportions, the head of a child carries a greater proportion of the body weight than in the adult, which predisposes them to pressure related tissue injury over the occiput.

Drug Reactions

A severe acute cutaneous reaction to drugs is perhaps the second most commonly encountered entity in the critically ill. The fact that patients in the ICU generally undergo polypharmacy, makes it difficult to pinpoint the culprit. In addition, a lot of cutaneous reactions to drugs may mimic primary disorders of the skin with similar clinical presentation. A French study has shown that these reactions may account for up to 19% of adverse reactions in hospitalized patients. Another cohort study has put the incidence at around 11%. Antimicrobials are the drugs most commonly incriminated followed by nonsteroidal anti-inflammatory drugs. Cutaneous reaction patterns due to drugs may vary from life-threatening ones to less serious rashes.

Acute cutaneous drug reactions (ACDR) can be classified as:

- Severe ACDRs—angioedema, anaphylaxis, Stevens-Johnson syndrome—toxic epidermal necrolysis (SJS-TEN), DRESS syndrome, erythroderma.
- Other less severe ACDRs—lichenoid eruptions, acneiform lesions, erythema nodosum, fixed drug eruptions, exanthems.

The severe ACDRs have been dealt in detail in other sections. The latter category might be encountered in the ICU but is unlikely to be a primary cause for an admission. However, it is important for the nurse working in the ICU to be aware that these eruptions can result from drugs and the basic skin care has to be tailored to match the condition.

Some common basic principles of nursing care that apply to all drug reactions are as follows:

- Vigilance and keen inspection of the skin on a daily basis; this should be carried out in good light and any observation is noted in the case records.
- Progress of rash; most rashes associated with drug reactions tend to develop quickly and might change the morphology rapidly. These changes must be carefully observed and action taken at the earliest sign of these turning serious.
- A good history to establish a temporal correlation with a drug is essential. These must include any 'over the counter' formulations and medicines suggested by friends and family.

A special mention of angioedema resulting from drugs is important because of its life-threatening potential. Although, almost any drug can cause acute angioedema, the commonest category is the ACE inhibitors. This group of drugs includes benazepril, lisinopril, captopril, ramipril, enalapril, etc. Its onset requires immediate recognition and sometimes begins as wheals in other parts of the skin but may evolve rapidly to cause acute airway obstruction. Often it is the nurse who will be alone on duty and hence he/she needs to inform the on duty physician immediately and institute emergency management. Early recognition is the cornerstone of management of such situation.

Perineal Dermatitis

This entity causes considerable morbidity in patients who are incontinent and admitted in the ICU. The inflammation involves the perineal area, upper thigh and buttock and may range in severity from erythema to varying degrees of skin disruption. Because of the presence of urine, the pH of the skin in this area is increased resulting in impaired skin integrity. The rate of development of perineal dermatitis is much higher in patients with fecal incontinence. Perineal dermatitis also predisposes patients to urinary tract infection and pressure ulcers.

The first step in the care is to ensure that the patient is kept dry. Absorbent pads are important and must be changed at regular intervals. Dimethicone and other no-rinse cleansers are effective and best applied on disposable cloth and skin is wiped with these to remove feces and urine. Zinc oxide creams are effective barriers and have been used since a long time. The only challenge is removing the zinc cream especially when the skin is fragile or macerated. This requires expert nursing care skills and ICU nurses must be encouraged to protect the skin and not to wait till it breaks down.

Apart from these well-established entities, there are special nursing challenges in the critically ill. The fact that most of these patients are unable to care for themselves due to the severity of their illness, varying degrees of immobility, the presence of various life support equipment and medical or pharmacological paralysis, makes the job of the nurses more intensive. Some special aspects of managing these patients have been discussed below.

Oral Care Interventions

Patients in the ICU demand the highest standards of professional care. In the presence of more acute and life-threatening problems, oral care becomes a low priority and this is often neglected in the ICU. Organisms that colonize the mouth of critically ill patients have shifted from the naturally present gram positive flora to more virulent gram negative strains. These may find their way into the lower respiratory tract. Good oral hygiene can prevent this.

Assessment of the oropharynx on a daily basis is part of the routine nursing activity in ICU. However, in presence of intubation this can be a challenge. The presence of tubes and bite preventers can obstruct mouth care. Since dislodging of vital devices can cause death, nurses are generally reluctant to carry out oral hygiene procedures. The use of the 'BRUSHED Assessment model' has been found to be of great help in identifying oral problems by nurses. The gold standard in mouth care is the use of a toothbrush and a fluoride tooth paste.In a small minority of patients on anticoagulants, this should be done with utmost care, or avoided. The following protocol may be made a standard bedside instruction for all nurses:

- Wash hands and wear gloves.
- If patient is conscious, explain that the mouth will be cleaned.
- Using a soft pediatric brush and a pea size quantity of fluorinated paste, clean the teeth, gums and tongue.
- If a bite block is in place, remove it, clean and replace at the end of the cleaning procedure.
- Use a 10 ml syringe and a nonalcoholic mouthwash to rinse out the tooth paste and swab/suction it out.
- Apply petroleum jelly to the lips.

In cases where brushing is not possible, a gauze soaked in chlorhexidine mouthwash is effective in reducing plaque. This has been shown to have a bacteriostatic action for about 12 hours against gram positive and negative bacteria, yeasts and fungi.

Eye Care Interventions

Patients in acute care environments are likely to have impaired protective mechanisms. The risk is particularly high in unconscious and sedated patients. Like oral care, eye care too, in a critically ill patient is of relatively low priority. All the same, simple nursing procedures are all that is required to prevent some serious damage to the eyes in patients admitted in ICU.

The normal blink reflex is deranged in sedated patients specially those on ventilators. Use of muscle relaxants is common in these patients and this further compromises the protective tear film coverage of the eye. In addition, inadequate eye closure also leads to increase in tear film evaporation. The end result is dry eyes leading to varying degrees of loss of corneal and conjunctival defenses. Immediate effects include superficial corneal abrasions and in the long run corneal ulcers are not unusual.

Some simple nursing interventions to prevent these complications include:
- Maintain eye hygiene by cleansing the eyes with gauze dipped in normal saline.
- Use methylcellulose eye drops as artificial tears at regular intervals.
- Passive eye closure using gauze and adhesive tape.
- Eye shields.

Some studies have shown that using swimming goggles and regular moisturization of the eyes with gauze soaked in saline is more efficacious than the use of lubricants and tape.

NURSING CARE OF THE SKIN IN DERMATOLOGICAL EMERGENCIES

There are a few skin conditions that are acute, life-threatening and associated with significant mortality. There is disruption of the skin structure and function leading to widespread impact on various functions of the skin including temperature regulation, fluid balance, barrier function, metabolic and nutritional functions. A cohesive medical and nursing team is indispensible for an eventual successful outcome in these patients.

Stevens-Johnson Syndrome–Toxic Epidermal Necrolysis

This disease spectrum represents the most commonly encountered example of life-threatening skin disease. SJS–TEN is an acute hypersensitivity reaction to a drug or sometimes to a bacterial, viral or fungal infection. The largest study on medications related to SJS-TEN pointed towards sulphonamides, anticonvulsants and certain non-steroidal anti-inflammatory drugs as the common causative agents. The result is widespread epidermal necrosis leading to itching, burning, skin tenderness and finally dusky erythema leading on to sheets of denuded skin. This leads to massive fluid loss, electrolyte imbalance, superadded infection, impaired temperature regulation and excessive energy consumption. Involvement of the mucous membrane is severe leading to cicatricial sequelae on healing. Mortality may vary from between 10% in SJS to 35% in TEN.

A specific score (SCORTEN) uses a seven point system scored as 1 in the presence of a parameter and 0 in its absence. The scores are assessed every 3 days to prognosticate the patient. A low score of 0 to 1 is associated with low mortality of 3.2%, 2 points with 12.2 %, 3 points with 35.8%, 4 points with 58.3% and >5 points with >90% mortality.

The first step is immediate withdrawal of the offending drug. The second step is intensive and specialized nursing care of the skin. Dedicated nursing for 24 hours with one nurse for one or a maximum of two such patients at any given time is crucial for better outcome. This contributes significantly to a low mortality.

There are both general and specific nursing interventions:

General Nursing Interventions

- Maintain environmental temperature around 30° to 32° C.
- Careful aseptic handling of patient.
- Venous lines for peripheral access should be as far away from the affected skin as possible.
- Careful and accurate intravenous fluid correction.
- Regular monitoring of blood sugar levels.
- Avoid use of adhesive tapes and other dressing material.
- In case of severe oropharyngeal ulceration, feeding through a nasogastric tube.
- Catheterization to avoid pain during micturition and consequent retention.
- Pain and anxiety relief.

Specific Nursing Interventions

- *Skin care:* No consensus exists on whether the denuded epidermis should be retained or debrided. However, most centers follow a conservative approach and leave it in place as natural dressing. In order to protect this exposed epithelium, clean, sterile and non-adhesive dressings such as gauze impregnated with petrolatum jelly, silver nitrate or povidone iodine must be loosely draped over the body. Adhesive tapes must always be avoided. Some centers are now using biologic covers such as cadaveric allograft and autologus epidermal sheets, after epidermal stripping.

  Patients should be bathed daily very gently and all open areas monitored for signs of secondary infection.

- *Genital care:* This part is often missed while nursing acutely damaged skin. It is important to highlight the fact that two opposing denuded mucosal surfaces, as in the vulva and prepuce, are very prone to healing with adhesions. Therefore, the nurse must take special care to maintain good hygiene in these areas and use non-adhesive dressings to allow healing to occur. Daily examination of genitalia and breaking down early adhesions is imperative.

- *Mouth care:* Most of these patients have severe oral erosions that are not only painful but also prevent feeding. Use of regular medicated mouthwash 3 to 4 times a day followed by the application of antifungal oral paint is important. Petrolatum jelly gauze applied to the lips helps to prevent formation of adhesions on healing. In milder cases, who are on liquid diets orally, local analgesics and anesthetics may be used prior to feeding.
- *Eye care:* This requires specialist help because the damage can range from mild to severe. In its worst form corneal ulcers may develop resulting in loss of eye sight. Early advice and follow-up by an ophthalmologist may prevent sequel like adhesions. In terms of general measures, nurses must help the entire range of eye movements in every patient and use bland, lubricating eye drops.
- *Nutrition:* The energy and protein requirements of these patients who are in a hyper-catabolic state are directly proportional to the body surface area involved. A liquid diet is most advisable for patients with dysphagia. The aim of nursing such patients is to ensure that adequate calorie intake is maintained through the use of soft, smooth food and parenteral/nasogastric feeding is delayed or avoided as far as possible. However, a careful watch and calculation of calorie intake is important to make the decision to switch over to nasogastric feeding, if required.
- *Fluid intake:* Fluid loss in patients with SJS-TEN can be significant due to increased insensible loss. A careful input output chart is essential. Dehydration and renal impairment are not unusual in these patients and thus fluid monitoring is crucial. Intravenous lines may be a source of infection and must be changed and observed regularly. Oral fluid intake in the range of 100 to 200 ml must be encouraged since it also keeps the esophagus clean and patent.
- *Pain management:* The experience of pain and its management must be individualized. The use of pain relief also depends on the available resources for monitoring. It is, of course, preferable to keep the patient awake and conscious. But if the skin involvement is severe, it might become necessary to sedate the patient. Long acting moderate potency opioid drugs are good for persistent pain whilst short acting ones are effective when given before procedures. Some patients require anxiolytics, especially as a pre-procedure measure.
- *Rehabilitation:* Patients who have had SJS-TEN require ongoing emotional support to explain the cause of their condition. Family members must be involved in all such counseling sessions. Early mobilization is the key to healing and prevention of contractures. Nurses must encourage patients to sit in chairs and start walking as soon as the skin condition allows.
- *Medical alert:* The patient must be made aware of the causative drug and the medical records should carry an alert about the causative drug in bold. In addition, the family members must also be informed about this hypersensitivity of the patient.

Expert and dedicated nursing plays a crucial role in positive outcome of these patients.

Epidermolysis Bullosa

This group of inherited disorders results in blistering of the skin due to routine handling of the infant and minor trauma. There are several types of epidermolysis bullosa (EB) based on the severity and level of separation in the skin layers. These are broadly classified into three types: EB simplex where separation is intraepidermal, junctional EB where the split is in the lamina lucida and the severest form of dystrophic EB where the separation is suprabasal.

Most of these infants have blistering at or soon after birth. In the less severe forms, education of the mother and family about care of the fragile skin is the primary aim but in the more severe dystrophic forms, the infant may need admission to a neonatal intensive care unit.

The aims of caring infants with epidermolysis bullosa EB:
- Protection of skin against trauma, even the mildest.
- Prevention of secondary infection.
- Maintaining general nutrition.
- Minimizing deformity.
- Avoiding formation of contractures.
- Empowering parents and caregivers through transfer of knowledge and skills to care the infant in future.

Following are the general principles of skin care of the children with EB:

- *Skin protection*: Skin in epidermolysis bullosa is very fragile. Common day to day frictional stresses that do not affect normal skin can cause severe blistering in these patients. Prevention of blistering may be impossible but some daily interventions in child care routine can go a long way in reducing the occurrence of lesions and severity.
- *Bathing:* This can be one of the greatest challenges for the care-giver. Bathing is crucial to keep the skin clean, prevent infection, remove dead skin and crusts and remove adherent dressings. Babies can be soaked in a small tub/bath. Older children may prefer a shower. In all circumstances no force should be used to remove any stuck-on dressing. A medicated wash or addition of household bleach (2 tsp household bleach to 3.8 liters/1 gallon) to bath water may be used for asepsis.
- *Moisturizing:* Dry skin is itchy, therefore, it is important to use copious amounts of lotions or creams to keep the skin moist in these patients. Additionally, moist skin is less likely to split and crack.
- *Clothing:* Loose clothings made of soft, breathable fabric, should be worn inside out so that the seams do not rub against the skin. Avoid hurried undressing to prevent friction against head and ears.

- *Diapers:* It is better to use absorbent padding or cloth in place of conventional diapers with adhesive bands on the sides. Alternatively, cotton wool may be placed under the adhesive bands at sites of maximum contact and rubbing. It is important to keep the child dry at all times and avoid any maceration.
- *Bed linen:* These children are best placed on very soft, used and worn out cotton fabric in place of sheets. If available, satin sheets are a good option.
- *Shoes:* Both, too well fitting or too loose shoes can create friction resulting in blistering. One size loose shoes with comfortable access and a wide fit to accommodate extra padding are best suited for these children. However, despite best efforts, knees and toes in crawling babies and older children are the most trauma-prone areas.
- *Bandaging:* This is important because it helps to prevent further trauma, reduces the pain of existing wounds, helps to provide a moist environment for wound healing, and prevents secondary infection. Bandaging of non-wounded skin additionally prevents further trauma and blistering. Research in this field has resulted in great advances in the dressings available for EB but the principles underlying their usage are the same. The bandaging must be layered with the first layer in contact with the skin being nonadherent. The second layer should be of absorbent material, usually a type of gauze that is soft and protective at the same time. No adhesive tapes must ever be used on EB skin. No gloves must be used while dressing because they tend to stick to skin and can cause more damage.
- *Prevention of secondary infection:* Blistered skin is prone to infection. All oozing or moist sites are potentially prone to get infected. Applying topical antibiotics to gauze and placing it over the blister, rather than trying to rub in an ointment or cream, is less traumatizing. Bandaging helps to keep the dressing in place as well as provides protection. Minimize contamination of surfaces in touch with dressing material and keep hands clean.

Pemphigus Vulgaris and Other Bullous Dermatoses

Patients with these skin conditions do not routinely present as an acute emergency. Some neglected or mismanaged patients may, however, need specialized emergency care. Most of these cases are often secondarily infected and so relevant investigations followed by immediate institution of appropriate topical and systemic antibiotic therapy is important. The nurse must be competent in identifying early side effects of immunosuppressant drugs which are the cornerstone of treatment of these patients. Unlike SJS-TEN, these cases are chronic with a significant potential for relapse. Therefore, patients and their caregivers must be educated in self-care and regular follow-up. The other principles of nursing the affected skin are similar to those in SJS-TEN.

Erythroderma

In this group of conditions, most commonly secondary to psoriasis, atopic eczema, drug reactions or malignancies, the skin is covered with diffuse scaling. The loss of skin integrity has far reaching effects on the various functions of the skin. Due to increased blood flow to the skin, function of previously compromised heart may be severely affected. Thermoregulation is altered with patients experiencing chills and rigors. Severe itching seriously compromises the barrier function of the skin making it very prone to secondary infections.

Nursing Interventions

- Keep the room temperature between 30° to 32° C.
- Bathe the patient daily with a pH matched soap substitute to prevent drying out of the skin. Addition of a bath additive may help.
- Use of occlusive dressings and wet wraps helps to reduce inflammation and pruritus.
- Generous use of emollients 3 to 4 times a day helps to soothe the skin whilst providing a barrier to secondary infection. The emollient must be applied right after a bath in order to trap the moisture soaked during bathing.
- Patient must be given a regular manicure to prevent damage from scratching.
- Soft, breathable fabric that is nonirritating to the skin must be used.
- Any sign of secondary infection as indicated by erythema or increased local temperature must be noted and appropriate antibiotics instituted.
- A high protein, high calorie diet must be instituted to prevent hypoalbuminemia and its consequences. This will have to be continued even after discharge and so family members must be instructed about diet.

In conclusion, prompt recognition of conditions leading to potentially fatal acute skin failure, and its aggressive and intensive specialized management, as for any other organ failure, can significantly prevent morbidity and mortality. Dermatologists must take lead in highlighting the presence of this as yet under estimated entity, the "acute skin failure". Nurses must be trained in providing specialized care of skin in such conditions ensuring a positive patient outcome.

SUGGESTED FURTHER READING

1. Bastuji-Garin S, Fouchard N, Bertocchi N, Roujeau JC, Revuz J, Wolkenstein P. SCORTEN: a severity-of-illness score for toxic epidermal necrolysis. J Invest Dermatol 2000;115:149–53.

2. Bours G, DeLaat E, Halfens R, Lubbers M. Prevalence, risk factors and prevention of pressure ulcers in Dutch intensive care units. Intensive Care Med 2001;27:1599–1605.
3. Campos-Fernandez Mdel M, Ponce-De-Leon-Rosales S, Archer-Dubon C, Orozco-Topete R. Incidence and risk factors for cutaneous adverse drug reactions in an intensive care unit. Rev Invest Clin 2005;57:770–4.
4. Chikoti M, Lehloenya R, Wallace J. Management of Stevens-Johnson syndrome and toxic epidermal necrolysis in a low resourced setting. Community Dermatology 2011;7:17–32.
5. Cox J. Predictors of pressure ulcers in adult critical care patients. Am J Crit Care 2011;20:364–75.
6. Eachempati S, Hydo L, Barie P. Factors influencing the development of decubitus ulcers in critically ill surgical patients. Crit Care Med 2001;29:1678–82.
7. George Susannah MC, Harrison David A, Welch Catherine A, Nolan Kathleen M, Friedmann Peter S. Dermatological conditions in intensive care: a secondary analysis of the Intensive Care National Audit & Research Centre (ICNARC) Case mix programme database. Critical Care 2008;12 Suppl 1:S1.
8. Ghislain PD, Roujeau JC. Treatment of severe drug reactions: Stevens-Johnson syndrome, toxic epidermal necrolysis and hypersensitivity syndrome. Dermatol Online J 2002;8(1):5.
9. Gray M, Ratliff C, Donovan A. Perineal skin care for the incontinent patient. Adv Skin Wound Care 2002;15:170–8.
10. Gray M. Preventing and managing perineal dermatitis: a shared goal for wound and continence care. J Wound Ostomy Continence Nurs 2004;31(1 suppl):S2-S9.
11. Green T, Manara AR, Park GR. Dermatological conditions in the intensive care unit. Hosp Update 1989;15:367–76.
12. Hayes J, Jones C. A collaborative approach to oral care during critical illness. Dent Health 1995;34:6–10.
13. Hennessey TD. Some antibacterial properties of chlorhexidine. J Periodontal Res 1973;8:61–7.
14. Irvine C. Skin Failure: a real entity: discussion paper. J R Soc Med 1991; 84:412–3.
15. Keller P, White J, van Ramshorst B, van der Werken C. Pressure ulcers in intensive care patients: a review of risks and prevention. Intensive Care Med 2002;28:1379–88.
16. Langemo DK, Brown G. Skin fails too: acute, chronic, and end stage skin failure. Adv Skin Wound Care 2006;19:206–11.
17. Lehloenya R. Management of Stevens-Johnson syndrome and toxic epidermal necrolysis. Curr Allergy Clin Immunol 2007;20:124–8.
18. Longhurst RH. A cross sectional study of the oral health care instructions given to nurses during their basic training. Br Dent J 1998;184:453–7.
19. Ly L, Su JC. Dressings used in epidermolysis bullosa blister wounds: a review. J Wound Care 2008;17:482, 484–6.
20. Nix DH. Validity and reliability of Perineal assessment tool. Ostomy Wound Manage 2002;48:43–9.

21. Pasek TA, Geyser A, Sidoni M, Harris P, Warner J, Spence A, et al. Skin care team in the pediatric intensive care unit: A model for excellence. Crit Care Nurse 2008;28:125–35.
22. Roujeau JC, Kelly JP, Naldi L, Rzany B, Stern RS, Anderson T, et al. Medication use and the risk of Stevens-Johnson syndrome or toxic epidermal necrolysis. N Engl J Med 1995;333:1600–7.
23. Roujeau JC, Stern RS. Severe adverse cutaneous reactions to drugs. N Engl J Med 1994.331;1272–85.
24. Ryan TJ. Disability in dermatology. Br J Hosp Med 1991;46:33–6.
25. Schindler CA, Mikhailov TA, Kuhn EM, Christopher J, Conway P, Ridling D, et al. Protecting fragile skin: nursing interventions to decrease development of pressure ulcers in pediatric intensive care. Am J Crit Care 2011;20:26–35.
26. Shannon ML, Lehman CA. Protecting the skin of the elderly patient in the intensive care unit. Crit Care Nurs Clin North Am 1996;8:17–28.
27. Sivasanker S, Jasper S, Simon S, Jacob P, John G, Raju R. Eye care in ICU. Indian J Crit Care Med 2006;10:11–4.
28. Solis I, Krouskop T, Trainer N, Marburger R. Supine interface pressure in children. Arch Phys Med Rehabil 1998;69:524–6.
29. Theaker C, Mannan M, Ives N, Soni N. Risk factors for pressure sores in the critically ill. Anesthesia 2000;55:221–4.
30. Treloar DM, Stechmiller JK. Use of a clinical assessment tool for orally intubated patients. Am J Crit Care 1995;4:355–60.
31. Willock J, Hughes J, Tickle S, Rossiter G, Johnson C, Pye H. Pressure sores in children: the acute hospice perspective. J Tissue viability 2000;10:59–62.

Dermatology Intensive Care Unit (DICU)

Arun C Inamadar

- Concept of intensive care and intensive care unit
- Admission criteria for DICU
- Multidisciplinary approach in patients admitted in DICU
- How to set up DICU?
- Instruments and equipments
- Emergency drugs
- Skills to be acquired by dermatologists

INTRODUCTION

The prototype diseases with acute skin failure, e.g. toxic epidermal necrolysis (TEN) and dermatological emergency, e.g. pustular psoriasis are conventionally managed in 'burn centers' and 'general intensive care units' respectively. In some centers even today there is no provision to isolate these patients from others. A better understanding of the systemic effects of skin diseases and multidisciplinary approach to handle such situations has generated the idea of setting up dermatology intensive care units (DICU), at least in tertiary care hospitals.

CONCEPT OF INTENSIVE CARE AND INTENSIVE CARE UNIT

Intensive care implies close monitoring and constant medical care of patients with life-threatening conditions or critical illnesses. Intensive care unit is a specialized section of a hospital designed and equipped to provide comprehensive continuous care of critically ill patients who may benefit from treatment.

Intensive care unit (ICU) can be set up to provide specialized care to patients with a range of specific conditions like cardiac ICU, neuro-medical ICU, pediatric ICU, neonatal ICU, etc.

Do Patients with Dermatological Illnesses Really Need Intensive Care and Dermatology Intensive Care Unit?

Emergency management is required for the patients suffering from dermatological diseases, which demand early diagnosis, hospitalization, long-term careful monitoring and multidisciplinary intervention.

Some patients with dermatological disorders may land up with acute skin failure (akin to cardiac failure or respiratory failure) and require special attention and management protocol. Skin is the prime barrier of human body and performs metabolic, endocrine and thermoregulatory functions. Extensive loss of skin makes a patient prone to develop complications like hypothermia, hypoproteinemia, dehydration, electrolyte imbalance and septicemia. These patients may have distinct signs and symptoms, which may be recognized and cared only by dermatologists. Patients with acute skin failure require a strictly aseptic environment because of the compromised skin barrier (physical as well as immunological). Optimum environmental temperature, adequate humidity and asepsis are the critical factors in their well-being. Some medical complications are commoner in these patients like any other seriously ill patient; these include, cardiac failure, pulmonary edema secondary to fluid overload, aspiration pneumonia, deep vein thrombosis and disseminated intravascular coagulation. Hence, it is appropriate to nurse and treat these patients in a separate set up, DICU, specially made for patients with acute skin failure.

ADMISSION CRITERIA FOR DICU

Intensive care has been demonstrated to improve the outcome in severely ill and unstable patients. Decisions on DICU admission are based on the diagnosis of 'dermatological emergencies' and on expected complications of the condition. A list of dermatological emergencies has been presented in chapter 1 (Table 1.2). Not all these conditions require admission to DICU; some of them can be managed in general ICU because of predominant systemic involvement (e.g. purpura fulminans, anaphylactic shock, meningococcemia, dengue shock syndrome, etc.); others may be managed in dermatology ward with close monitoring for signs of deterioration, so that they may be transferred to DICU, if necessity arises (e.g. leprosy reactions, acute urticaria with angioedema, erythroderma without complication, etc.). Hence, it is the patients with acute skin failure (severe adverse cutaneous drug reactions, immunobullous and mechanobullous disorders, acute generalized pustular psoriasis, erythroderma with complications, etc.), who require immediate admission to DICU.

MULTIDISCIPLINARY APPROACH IN PATIENTS ADMITTED IN DICU

Multidisciplinary care is mandatory for managing dermatological emergencies. It was appropriately said by Dr Jorizzo *(Professor of Deramatology, Wake-Forest University School of Medicine, Winston-Salem, NC, USA)*, 'in most cases of a true cutaneous emergency, the patient needs to be managed jointly, where the dermatologist is the advisor. We are very good at co-managing patients with lots of input to other specialists.'

When intervention of various specialties is required to manage difficult cases, it is important to talk to the other specialists of the treating team personally rather than writing notes or reading written notes; it helps to undertake important decisions regarding patient management by mutual exchange of ideas as well as maintain a professional relationship with others.

HOW TO SET UP DICU?

The primary requirements to set up a DICU are:

- Space
- Equipments
- Specific instruments
- Emergency drugs
- Management protocols for each of the common conditions
- Charts for easy and uniform display of the management strategies
- Books for quick reference.

Subsequently, following arrangements are to be done:

- Constitution of DICU team: The team should consist of dermatologist, physician, pediatrician, anesthetist, surgeon, on-duty resident doctors and trained nurses. All members of the team must be conversant (either to perform or to assist) with the basic life support procedures and universal precautions.
- Rooms: It should be easily accessible from other ICUs, preferably established in the same complex. There must be minimum 5 rooms (for patients, on-duty doctors, waiting room with lockers for attendees, store-room and toilet).
- Number of beds: Up to four beds are ideal in consideration with the load of the cases.
- Sterilization facility.
- Provisions for maintenance of asepsis by following measures:
  - Handwash with antiseptic solution.
  - Use of gloves while handling the patient.

- Use of sterile gowns, caps and masks, before doctors, nurses or other health care workers enter the DICU.
- Total restriction of entry inside the DICU with footwear and other personal items.
• Facilities for all conducting procedures and basic life support measures.
• Provisions for regular disinfection of the DICU.

A dermatology intensive care unit (DICU) set up has been displayed in **Figures 7.1** and **7.2**.

INSTRUMENTS AND EQUIPMENTS

Instruments and equipments required to set up DICU can be categorized into five groups:

Group I: Patient monitoring equipments
Group II: Diagnostic equipments
Group III: Life support and resuscitation equipments
Group IV: Consumables
Group V: Others

A list of necessary instruments and equipments has been presented in **Table 7.1**. In case of nonavailability of air conditioning machine, room humidifiers (air cooler) and room heaters may be used temporarily.

Use of waterbed or air-fluidized bed for critically ill patients admitted in DICU helps to prevent development of pressure sores.

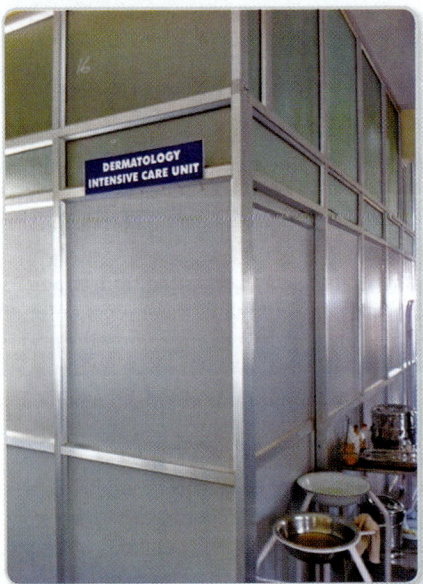

Figure 7.1: A DICU chamber in the author's department

Dermatology Intensive Care Unit (DICU)

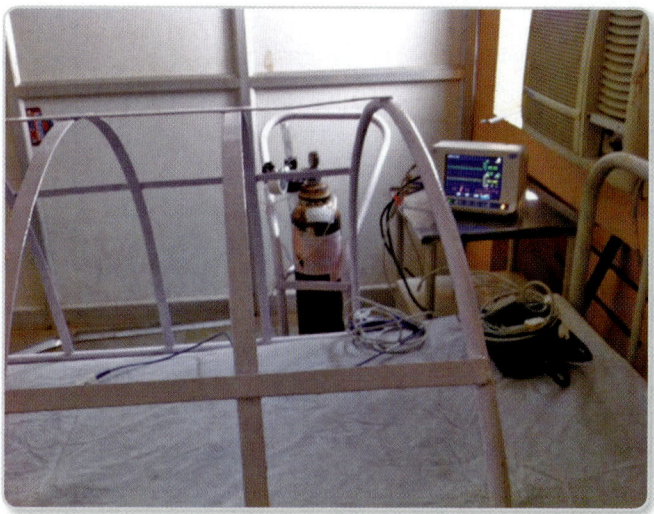

Figure 7.2: A patient's bed in DICU chamber with burn cage, oxygen cylinder and bedside multi-parameter monitor

Table 7.1: List of instruments and equipments required to set up DICU

Group I	Patient monitoring equipments	– Sphygmomanometer – Pulse oximeter – Cardiac monitor – ECG machine – Blood gas analyzer – Thermometer (oral and rectal)
Group II	Diagnostic equipments	– Glucometer – Kits for various spot tests – Portable X-ray machine – Sterile test tubes/bottles for collection of microbiological samples
Group III	Life support and resuscitation equipments	– Defibrillator – Laryngoscope – Endotracheal tube – Mask and resuscitation bag – Oxygen cylinder – Oxygen inhalation mask with tubing – Nebulizer with mask – Suction machine – Emergency medication box – Mechanical ventilator

Contd...

Contd...

Group IV	Consumables	– IV cannula – IV fluid transfusion and blood transfusion sets – Central venous catheter – Arterial catheter – Central venous catheterization set – Tourniquets – Venesection set – Disposable syringe and needles – Ryle's tube – Foley's catheter – Tongue spatula – Condom (for urinary drainage of male patients) – Uro-bag with connecting tubes – Dressing material – Eye pads – Vaseline gauze – Methylated spirit – Povidone iodine – Normal saline – Hydrogen peroxide – Adhesive tape – Torch/focus light
Group V	Others	– Air-conditioner OR room humidifier and room heater – Air fluidized bed/water bed – IV fluid stand – Burn cage – McIntosh sheet

Waterbed/water mattress/floatation bed is made up of soft polyvinyl chloride (PVC) or similar material and is provided with single or interconnected flow chambers to fill it with water. Modern waterbeds have interconnected air and fluid chambers. Waterbeds may be warmed with additional thermostatic control and it may be set at body temperature or according to patient's comfort level. When in use, waterbed is shaped around patient's body to minimize pressure especially over joints and spine. However, it has certain disadvantages like:

- Patient may feel uncomfortable due to sensation of floating.
- Water bed with temperature regulation system may result in dysregulation of body temperature and dehydration in patients with acute skin failure.
- Troubleshooting like accidental leakage.

Frequent posture change of the patient has to be continued even if water bed/air fluidized bed is used.

EMERGENCY DRUGS

Emergency drug tray should be kept ready all the time. Care must be taken to check the expiry dates of the stored drugs and to replace them regularly. Following is the list of drugs which need to be kept in DICU:

A. **Cardiovascular and hemodynamic drugs:**
   - Symapathomimetics: Adrenaline, dopamine, dobutamine
   - Diuretic: Frusemide
   - Atropine
   - Colloids and crystalloids
   - Anticoagulants: Heparin, low molecular weight heparin
   - Fibrinolytic agents: Streptokinase, urokinase

B. **Acid base balance and correction of electrolytes:**
   Sodium bicarbonate, Calcium chloride, Calcium gluconate

C. **Respiratory drugs:**
   - Aminophylline
   - Nebulization with bronchodilators (salbutamol)

D. **Others:**
   - Hydrocortisone, ampoules of 25% dextrose

Discussion about use of these drugs related to dermatological emergencies has been included in chapters 2 and 9. Some of the drugs to be kept in DICU for emergency situations, has been displayed in **Figure 7.3**.

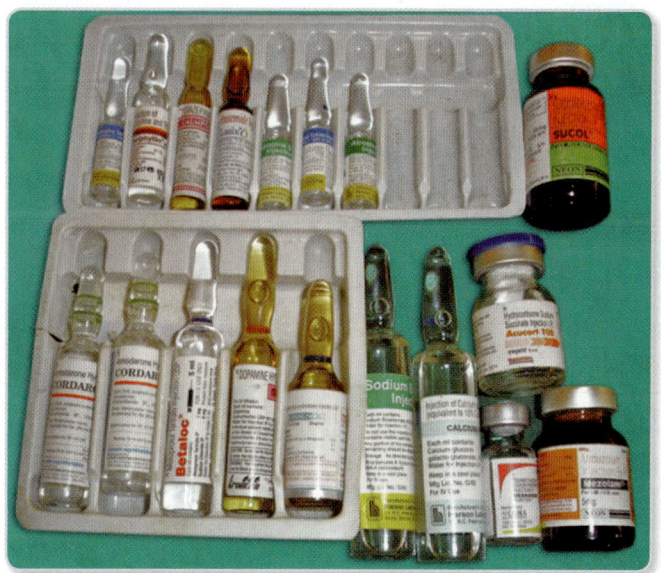

Figure 7.3: Emergency drugs to be kept in DICU *(Courtesy:* Prof DG Talikoti, Anesthetist, Bijapur)

Protocols and Charts

Ready protocols and displayed charts are handy to deal the emergency situations even by resident doctors attending the case and uniformity of management of cases is maintained. These protocols must be revised regularly at par with recent developments in the subject and according to the standard practice followed in other premier institutions. Ready protocols are required mainly regarding the following:

- Management of anaphylaxis
- Fluid and electrolyte therapy
- Steps of cardiopulmonary resuscitation
- Management of cardiac failure
- Management of respiratory failure
- Management of hypotension (shock)
- Heparinization
- Nutritional therapy.

Certain charts of importance in relation to dermatological emergencies are to be specially prepared and displayed. Following are the examples of few such charts:

- Causes of acute skin failure
- Complications of acute skin failure
- Indications of antibiotics in acute skin failure
- SCORTEN
- List of drugs causing severe cutaneous drug reactions
- Calculation of body surface area (adults and children)
- Drug dosage (adults and children)
- Calculation of drug dosage in special situations (hepatic failure, renal failure).

SKILLS TO BE ACQUIRED BY DERMATOLOGISTS

Dermatologists should be ready to undertake certain emergency maneuvers as a basic physician and also in case the required specialist is not able to reach DICU in specific time period. Below is the list of skills to be acquired by the dermatologists:

- Insertion of IV cannula
- Ryles' tube insertion
- Urinary catheterization
- Endotracheal intubation
- Venesection
- Central venous catheterization
- Basic life support and emergency resuscitation.

In conclusion, establishment of DICU can change the way dermatologists can manage critically ill patients effectively. This extra step may increase the life expectancy of patients with Stevens-Johnson syndrome, toxic epidermal necrolysis, acute generalized pustular psoriasis, pemphigus, etc, and the outlook of this specialty may revert to as a dynamic subject.

SUGGESTED FURTHER READING

1. Bastuji-Garin S, Fouchard N, Bertocchi M, Roujeau JC, Revuz J, Wolkenstein P. SCORTEN: a severity-of-illness score for toxic epidermal necrolysis. J Invest Dermatol 2000;115:149–53.
2. Davidovici BB, Wolf R. Emergencies in dermatology: Diagnosis, classification and therapy. Expert Rev Dermatol 2007;2:549–62.
3. Hettiaratchy S, Moloney D, Clarke J. Patients with acute skin loss: are they best managed on a burns unit? Ann R Coll Surg Engl 2001;83: 26–9.
4. Inamadar AC, Palit A. Acute skin failure: concept, causes, consequences and care. Indian J Dermatol Venereol Leprol 2005;71:379–85.

chapter 8

Drugs Used in Dermatological Emergencies

Arun C Inamadar, Abhay Mani Martin

- Classification
- Adrenaline
- Dopamine
- Dobutamine
- Frusemide
- Atropine
- Colloids and crystalloids
- Sodium bicarbonate
- Calcium gluconate
- Oxygen therapy
- Corticosteroids
- Cyclosporine
- Methotrexate
- Cyclophosphamide
- Vincristine

INTRODUCTION

Emergency situations arising out of dermatological illnesses are relatively rare. However, when such cases are encountered, the clinician has to be ever vigilant and therapy should be started early to reduce morbidity and mortality. A working knowledge of life saving drugs used in such situations is crucial for successful outcome in management. The following section deals with the common drugs used in the management of dermatological emergencies.

CLASSIFICATION

Drugs employed in dermatologic emergencies may be categorized as follows:

Drugs Used to Overcome the Critical Condition of a Patient

- *Cardiovascular and hemodynamic drugs:*
    - Sympathomimetics: Adrenaline, dopamine, dobutamine
    - Diuretic: Frusemide
    - Atropine

Drugs Used in Dermatological Emergencies

  - Colloids and crystalloids
  - Anticoagulants: Heparin, low molecular weight heparin
  - Fibrinolytic agents: Streptokinase, urokinase
- *Acid base balance and correction of electrolytes:*
   Sodium bicarbonate, calcium chloride, calcium gluconate
- *Respiratory drugs:*
  - Aminophylline
  - Nebulization with bronchodilators (salbutamol)
- *Others:*
  - Hydrocortisone
  - Dextrose (25% ampoules)
  - Oxygen therapy

Drugs Used for Definitive Treatment of a Dermatological Condition Giving Rise to Dermatological Emergency

- Corticosteroids
- Intravenous immunoglobulin (IVIG)
- Immunosuppressives
  - Cyclosporine
  - Methotrexate
  - Cyclophosphamide
- Vincristine

In the following section, indications, contraindications and use of these agents (relevant to dermatological emergency only) will be discussed.

ADRENALINE

Indications

Sudden cardiac arrest, anaphylaxis, severe acute urticaria, life-threatening angioedema, air-borne/contact urticaria, drug-induced urticaria, bites/stings/envenomations.

Dose

Standard dose – 0.01 mg/kg, high dose – 0.1 mg to 0.2 mg/kg.
(1:10000 = 0.1 mg/ml, 1:1000= 1.0 mg/ml.)
In angioedema and anaphylaxis, following dose is used:

Adults

Injection adrenaline is given subcutaneously, 0.3 to 0.5ml (1:1000 dilution), very slowly over 5 to 10 minutes. This may be repeated if necessary at an interval of 20 to 30 minutes. The injection has to be administered with an insulin syringe or 26G needle.

Children

A dosage of 0.1 mg/ml is recommended for the above indications.
No dosage modification is required in special situations like hepatic or renal failure.

Adverse Effects

Angina, anxiety, cardiac arrhythmias, dizziness, dyspnea, flushing, headache, hypertension, nausea, nervousness, sweating, tachycardia, vasoconstriction, vomiting, weakness.

Contraindications

- Absolute contraindication is in patients with asthma
- Organic heart disease or cardiac dilatation
- Closed-angle glaucoma

Precaution

Concomitant diseases like cerebrovascular insufficiency, heart disease, angina, hypertension, thyroid disorder and prostatic hypertrophy may increase the risk of epinephrine induced systemic effects. Old age and pregnancy may also enhance such risk.

Drug Interactions

Antihistamines (chlorpheniramine and diphenhydramine) may potentiate the sympathomimetic effects of adrenaline. Certain drugs, when used along with, may alter pharmacodynamic and pharmacokinetics of adrenaline. Caution should be taken while using the following drugs:
- Digitalis, mercurial diuretics, quinidine and other drugs which may sensitize the heart to arrhythmias.
- MAO-inhibitors or tricyclic antidepressants
- Concomitant use with some general anesthetics (chloroform, trichloroethylene, cyclopropane, halothane)

Prevention of Acute Adverse Effects and their Management

Adrenaline has to be administered with care only by experienced medical personnel. Symptoms like tachycardia, anxiety and nausea are usually self-limiting once the physiologic concentration of the drug is restored to its normal value. This occurs in about 20 to 30 minutes. However, there is a risk of cardiac arrest and acute vasoconstriction resulting in digital and limb gangrene. Strict supervision of dosage, concentration, dilution and route of administration of adrenaline in anaphylaxis is absolutely essential.

No specific antidote is available for accidental overdosage or wrong route of administration of adrenaline. Hence, caution in administration is the key to prevention of mishaps.

■ DOPAMINE

Indications

Patients with profound and persistent hypotension of any origin, patients in shock with or without acute renal shut down.

Dose

The available preparation contains 200 mg/5 ml;

- Low infusion rates (<10 µg/kg/min): Primarily β adrenergic effects, resulting in an increase in peripheral perfusion. Low dose is used in patients with poor renal perfusion.
- Higher infusion rates (>10 µg/kg/min): Primarily α adrenergic effect, causing peripheral vasoconstriction. This dose is used in patients with shock.

Adverse Effects

Subcutaneous leakage causes vasoconstriction and extravasation tissue necrosis.

Administration

Dopamine is stable for about 24 hours in sodium chloride or dextrose solution. It is given by continuous intravenous infusion.

■ DOBUTAMINE

It is primarily a β-1-adrenoceptor agonist and it has some α- agonist effect also. It is useful in cardiogenic shock (used with dopamine) and in low output heart failure, in the absence of hypertension. Dobutamine injection is available as 25 mg/ml, dose administered is 1 to 15 µg/kg/minute.

■ FRUSEMIDE

Indications

Heart failure, pulmonary edema, renal failure, peripheral edema.

Dose

- For the relief of edema dose is 20 to 120 mg/day orally; 20 to 40 mg IV/IM.

- For use in renal failure, 500 mg orally or 250 mg in 25 ml of IV fluid, administered as infusion (4 mg/minute).

Administration
Oral/intravenous injection/IV infusion/IM injection.

Adverse Effects
Nausea, pancreatitis and transient deafness associated with rapid IV infusion or injection, in patients with renal failure. There may be excess therapeutic effects in the form of electrolyte imbalance (hypokalemia, excess loss of magnesium and calcium) and hypotension due to low plasma volume.

Drug Interactions
Indomethacin reduces frusemide-induced diuresis.

ATROPINE

Atropine is a parasympatholytic agent. It reduces vagal tone, thus increasing the heart rate, and facilitating conduction through the bundle of His. It has no significant effect on peripheral blood vessels in therapeutic doses.

Indications
Atropine is useful in bradycardia following myocardial infarction, symptomatic bradycardia and heart block (neonatal LE). When used prophylactically before any invasive procedure, it may prevent vaso-vagal attack.

Dose
0.6 to 1.2 mg orally at night or 0.6 mg IV with maximum dose of 3 mg/day.

Contraindication
Not to be administered in patients with glaucoma and urinary retention.

COLLOIDS AND CRYSTALLOIDS

During emergency restoration of intravascular volume, it is more important to transfuse crystalloid solutions (isotonic saline), as it is immediately effective. However, these are excreted rapidly, without long-lasting effect. Colloids are macromolecules which remain in the circulation for longer period. Details of the usage of these agents have been discussed in chapter 3.

Crystalloids

Sodium is the major cation and determinant of osmotic pressure of the extracellular fluid. It is present in most crystalloid preparations as mixtures of sodium chloride and other physiologically active solutes. Crystalloid fluids are designed to expand the interstitial space and only 20% of these remain in the vascular space. Crystalloids are used:

- To replenish extracellular volume in dehydration
- For rapid volume replacement during hypotensive shock
- To maintain lifeline and basic hydration in a critically ill patient
- To administer drugs.

Following are the commonly used crystalloid solutions:

Normal Saline (0.9%)

It is isotonic to normal body fluid. It is the most common fluid used for rapid volume replenishment.

Ringer's Lactate

It is a balanced electrolyte solution that substitutes potassium and calcium for some of the sodium. Lactate is added as a buffer. When a critically ill patient is on long-term intravenous fluid therapy Ringer's Lactate may be used interchangeably with normal saline to replenish electrolytes. Extreme caution should be taken while using this fluid in patients with diabetes mellitus and renal failure.

Dextrose Solutions

It is available as:
- 5% dextrose solution (5% in water)
- 10% dextrose solution (10% in water)
- Dextrose saline (4% dextrose in 0.18% normal saline)

Dextrose solutions provide fluid without electrolytes and are source of calorie through carbohydrate source. One liter of 5% dextrose and 10% dextrose solution supplies approximately 170 kcal and 340 kcal respectively.

If calculation is not possible, typical daily maintenance fluid of a critically ill patient may be provided with infusion of 5% dextrose solution and normal saline up to a total volume of 2 liters.

Colloids

Colloidal solutions include dextrans (glucose polymer), gelatine (hydrolyzed collagen) and hydroxyethyl starch. These are large molecular weight substances which do not pass readily across capillary walls. The aim of using colloids is to expand the intravascular volume and to decrease the amount of fluid that leaves the intravascular space (plasma restoring effect/volume expanders). Adverse effects of colloids include anaphylactoid reactions. Commonly used colloids have been discussed below.

Dextran

These are synthetic colloids derived from the juice of sugar beets. The preparations are dextran-40 (mol. wt. 40,000) and dextran-70 (mol. wt. 70,000), available as 10% solutions. The rapid volume expansion achieved from infusion of dextran-40 is about twice the infused volume. It is sustained till 6 hours and > 50% is cleared thereafter. It may produce an anticoagulant effect as it inhibits platelet aggregation. Dextran-70 has also a plasma restoring effect for up to 5 to 6 hours and it is indicated to improve peripheral blood flow.

Human Serum Albumin

It may provide for about 80% of the colloidal osmotic pressure (COP) of plasma. The preparation is available as 5% (50 g/L) and 25% solution (250 g/L) in isotonic saline. The 5% solution has a COP of 20 mm Hg, whereas the 25% solution has a COP of 70 mm Hg. An infusion of 100 ml of 25% solution will expand the plasma volume to about 500 ml. The effect of albumin infusion persists for 24 to 36 hours. Dilutional coagulopathy may occur when large volume is used.

Characteristics of various intravenous fluids have been presented in Table 8.1

Table 8.1: Characteristics of various intravenous fluids

Contents	Ringer's lactate	Normal saline	Dextrose saline	Albumin (5%)
Na (mEq/L)	130	154	30	13–160
Cl (mEq/L)	109	154	30	130–160
Lactate mEq/L	28	0	0	0
Oncotic pressure mm Hg	0	0	0	20

■ SODIUM BICARBONATE

Indications

Metabolic acidosis and hyperkalemia.
It is available as 7.5% w/v, each ml contain 75 mg sodium bicarbonate.

Dose

For metabolic acidosis, the dose is 2 to 5 mEq/kg, IV infusion over 4 to 8 hours; for hyperkalemia the dose is 50 mEq IV, injected over 5 minutes.

Drug Interaction

It is precipitated with calcium in intravenous lines and inactivates catecholamines. Hence, IV line has to be flushed after administration of sodium bicarbonate, before administering other drugs.

CALCIUM GLUCONATE

Indication

Injection calcium gluconate is administered in patients with acute onset hypocalcemia.

Dose

It is administered as 10% solution, 10-20 ml, at the rate of about 2 ml/minute and followed by continuous IV infusion containing 40 ml/day with monitoring of plasma calcium.

Adverse Effects

Sudden and fatal cardiac arrest may occur with injection calcium gluconate. A premonitory sign of onset of adverse effect is a tingling sensation in the mouth and a feeling of warmth spreading over the body.

Heparin

Heparin is a sulfated mucopolyscchararide. It is a direct-acting anticoagulant. Heparin binds to antithrombin and this leads to rapid inhibition of the proteases of the coagulation pathway. The low molecular weight heparins (LMWH) are prepared from standard heparin by a variety of chemical techniques. Commercial preparations of LMWH contain various fractions and display different pharmacokinetics.

Intravenous and subcutaneous routes are preferred for administration, as heparin is poorly absorbed in the gastrointestinal tract. Monitoring therapy is by the activated partial thromboplastin time (APTT), the optimum therapeutic range being 1.5 to 2.5 times the control.

With the availability of cost effective and easy to monitor LMWH, there is widespread changes in the anticoagulation therapy. LMWH have become the preferred drugs for anticoagulation in deep vein thrombosis, prevention of thrombosis after myocardial infarction and postoperatively. Once daily subcutaneous administration is sufficient as the duration of action is longer than that of conventional heparin and no laboratory monitoring is required.

Indications and dose of heparin in various dermatological conditions requiring anticoagulation has been discussed in chapter 2.

Adverse effects include, bleeding, heparin-induced thrombocytopenia, osteoporosis, transient alopecia and hypersensitivity reactions, often noted with both heparin and LMWH.

OXYGEN THERAPY

Any patient admitted in dermatological intensive care unit with respiratory distress (dyspnea/tachypnea) or cyanosis must be administered 100% oxygen inhalation immediately. Patients with acute skin failure may develop adult respiratory distress syndrome (ARDS) as a complication and require oxygen inhalation. Other indications are septicemia, hypotensive shock, anaphylaxis and angioedema with laryngeal edema.

Before administering oxygen it must be humidified and warmed at optimal temperature (32°–37° C). This is specifically important in patients with endotracheal intubation where the oxygen is administered through the tube bypassing the normal physiological warming and humidification achieved in upper airway if it would have been administered through nasal route. Use of non-humidified and cool oxygen in infants <6 months may precipitate hypothermia.

CORTICOSTEROIDS

Indications

Indications of corticosteroids in dermatological emergencies are as follows:
- Acute or chronic urticaria and/or angioedema not responding to optimum dose of antihistamines.
- Severe cutaneous adverse drug reactions, like drug hypersensitivity syndrome; in some cases, in early stage of Stevens-Johnson syndrome.
- Vesiculobullous disorders.
- Life-threatening bites or envenomation.
- Erythroderma (nonpsoriatic).
- Kassabach-Merritt syndrome.

Corticosteroids Used in Emergency Care

- Hydrocortisone: Parenteral route; intravenous (IV) route preferred in acute emergencies. Administered in a dose of 25 to 100 mg, given IV.
- Betamethasone: Oral and parenteral.
- Dexamethasone: Oral and parenteral.
- Prednisolone: Oral, 0.5 to 1.0 mg/kg/day.
- Methylprednisolone: Oral, (available as 4 mg, 8 mg, 16 mg tablets) and parenteral.

Major Drug Interactions

- Carbamazepine, phenytoin, phenobarbital, rifampicin, rifabutin- decreases levels of prednisolone by affecting CYP3A4 metabolism.
- Clarithromycin, erythromycin, ketoconazole, itraconazole, oral contraceptives increase levels of prednisolone by affecting CYP3A4 metabolism.

- Action of insulin and oral hypoglycemics are opposed by the use of corticosteroids.

Dosage Schedule

Dosage schedule for corticosteroids (prednisolone) has been presented in **Table 8.2**. The usual recommended dosage in pediatric patients is 1 mg/kg daily initially and the dose is halved every 4 to 7 days.

Table 8.2: Dosage range for corticosteroids

High dosage	> 60 mg daily
Moderate dosage	40–60 mg daily
Low dosage	< 40 mg daily
Physiologic dose (replacement therapy)	5–7.5 mg daily

Adverse Effects

Short-term use of corticosteroids employed in emergency situations may result in following adverse effects:
- Gastritis, gastrointestinal hemorrhage.
- Headache and insomnia.
- Diabetes may be unmasked in susceptible individuals or diabetic individuals may develop hyperglycemia.
- Elevation of blood pressure may occur in hypertensive patients.

Rapid infusion of high dose corticosteroids (e.g. pulse therapy) may result in following adverse effects:
- Electrolyte shifts (hypokalemia and hypernatremia), leading to cardiac arrhythmias and sudden death.
- Anaphylactic reactions.
- Seizure.
- Acute psychosis.

Slower administration over 2 to 3 hours has minimized many of these serious side effects, and vital signs are to be monitored frequently. It is important to monitor serum electrolytes before and after steroid pulse therapy, particularly when patients are on concomitant treatment with diuretics.

Precaution

Caution should be taken in patients suffering from cirrhosis, ocular herpes simplex, hypertension, diabetes mellitus, congestive heart failure, diverticulitis, hypothyroidism, myasthenia gravis, osteoporosis, ulcerative colitis, psychiatric illness, renal insufficiency, and thromboembolic disorders. Latent tuberculosis may be reactivated; patients with positive tuberculin test should be monitored.

Clinical and Laboratory Monitoring

Protocol for clinical and laboratory monitoring during short-term corticosteroid therapy has been presented in **Table 8.3**. Monitoring guidelines for adverse effects of short-term corticosteroid therapy have been presented in **Table 8.4**.

Table 8.3: Protocol for patient monitoring during short course therapy with corticosteroids (< 3 weeks)

Category	Clinical examination	Lab monitoring
No preexisting co-morbidities (diabetes, asthma, hypertension)	• Watch for signs of infection or activation of septic foci • Monitor for weight gain	No specific laboratory monitoring required
Preexisting comorbidities		Blood sugar Blood pressure Serum triglyceride Serum potassium level

Table 8.4: Prevention and treatment of adverse effects due to short-term corticosteroid use

Adverse effects of short-term corticosteroid use	Prevention/treatment options
Hyperglycemia	– Monitor blood sugar – Oral hypoglycemic drugs/Insulin, as required – Expert consultation from physician or endocrinologist
Hypertension	– Monitor blood pressure – Administer antihypertensive
Acute gastritis/gastro-intestinal hemorrhage	– Preferably steroid is administered after meal/following feeding – Concurrent therapy with parenteral H-2 receptor blocker/proton pump inhibitor
Fluid overload	– Diuretics may be added
Electrolyte and acid base imbalance	– Monitoring of serum potassium regularly

INTRAVENOUS IMMUNOGLOBULIN

Intravenous immunoglobulin (IVIg) has been used in various dermatological conditions. Its use in dermatological emergencies is increasingly recognized. It is an effective and safe agent that can serve as an immunosuppressive and steroid-sparing agent.

Indications in Dermatological Emergency
- Toxic epidermal necrolysis
- Autoimmune bullous disorders like pemphigus
- Kawasaki disease

Contraindications
- IgA deficiency

Adverse Effects of IVIg Therapy and Prevention
Adverse effects related to IVIg therapy and the preventive measures have been presented in **Table 8.5**. Monitoring guidelines for IVIg therapy has been presented in **Table 8.6**.

Dosage Schedule
The most common dosage schedules of IVIg are:

Table 8.5: Adverse effects of IVIg therapy and preventive measures

Adverse effect	Features	Prevention
Infusion related adverse reactions	Fever, nausea, vomiting, headache, chills, low back ache, changes in blood pressure. These effects are mild and last half to one hour	Infusion rate slowed down or discontinued. Symptomatic management is advised with antihistamines and analgesics
Anaphylaxis	Notably in IgA deficiency with anti-IgA antibodies	Before starting therapy with IVIg, all patients must be screened for IgA deficiency
Fluid overload	Weight gain, edema. Occurs probably due to sucrose content in IVIg preparations	Patients with cardiac and renal disease need to be closely monitored
Hematological effects	Neutropenia, Hemolysis	Watch for ABO and Rh incompatibility
Neurological effects	Aseptic meningitis; presenting as headache, photophobia	Symptomatic treatment with analgesics and antiemetics, CSF analysis, if required
Thromboembolic events	Possibly because of changes in osmolality and serum viscosity. Cardiac and neurological thromboembolic phenomena	Slower rate of infusion at a lower dose

Table 8.6: Monitoring guidelines for IVIg therapy

Baseline
Clinical
• Complete history and physical examination.
• Assess for cardiac and renal risks
• Assess for fluid retention risk
Laboratory findings
• Complete blood count
• Liver and renal function tests
• Cardiac functional assay
• Immunoglobulin levels to exclude IgA deficiency
• Rheumatological work up
• RA factor, cryoglobulin, antineutrophil cytoplasmic antibody (ANCA) to assess renal risk with IVIg

Regimen A

1 to 2 g/kg/cycle divided into 3 equal doses, where each dose is given on each of the 3 consecutive days, i.e, 300 to 600 mg/kg/day for 3 days.

Regimen B

400 mg/kg/day given over a course of 5 consecutive days to constitute one cycle.

The infusion is given slowly over 4 to 4.5 hours. Close monitoring of vital signs and monitoring for adverse events and reactions is crucial. In patients with prior cardiac or renal disease, careful monitoring is required to prevent fluid overload.

CYCLOSPORINE

Cyclosporine A (CsA) is a potent immunosuppressive drug.

Indications and Contraindications

Cyclosporine may be employed in dermatologic emergencies like psoriatic erythroderma, acute generalized pustular psoriasis, vesiculobullous disorders and autoimmune urticaria. Contraindications of cyclosporine therapy have been presented in **Table 8.7.**

Dosage Schedule

Available formulations: Soft capsules, 25 mg, 50 mg and 100 mg. Used in acute-onset, unstable psoriasis at a dose of 3 to 5 mg/kg/day in two divided doses. In severe disease the drug may be started at highest dose (5 mg/kg/day) and thereafter reduced stepwise as disease is controlled.

Table 8.7: Contraindications of cyclosporine therapy

Absolute	Relative
• Impaired renal function • Uncontrolled hypertension • Hypersensitivity to CsA or any other ingredients in the formulation • Malignancy, even if it is clinically cured	• Controlled hypertension • Active infections • Concomitant methotrexate therapy • Pregnancy or lactation

Drug administration must be at a consistent time everyday following food. In critically ill patients it may be mixed in milk or orange juice to be administered through nasogastric tube.

Dose Adjustment in Special Situations

Renal Disease

Preexisting renal disease with significant renal dysfunction is an absolute contraindication for cyclosporine therapy. However, when cyclosporine is indicated in a patient with dermatologic emergency having moderate renal dysfunction, it would be wise to monitor serum creatinine levels closely (vide section on monitoring).

Hepatic Dysfunction

Metabolism of cyclosporine is primarily hepatic and hence monitoring of liver function tests is necessary when there is pre-existing liver disease. Further, cyclosporine is a potent enzyme inducer and caution should be taken while using hepatotoxic drugs concomitantly, e.g. methotrexate.

Hyperlipidemic Patients

Hyperlipidemia is a common adverse effect of cyclosporine A and it may aggravate preexisting hyperlipidemia. It is initially managed with dietary changes and later with lipid lowering drugs, if necessary.

Clinical and Laboratory Monitoring

The parameters to be monitored while the patient is on CsA therapy, have been presented in **Table 8.8**.

METHOTREXATE

Methotrexate (MTX) is a drug primarily used by oncologists and rheumatologists. Recently it has been in use for several chronic dermatoses. The only FDA-approved dermatological indication of MTX use is psoriasis.

Table 8.8: Monitoring schedule of a patient on CsA therapy

	Baseline	While on therapy
Clinical	PASI score Blood pressure Rule out active focus of infection including hepatitis B, C and tuberculosis Rule out malignancy	Twice daily record of blood pressure while admitted in hospital; Thereafter **Initial 3 months:** Every other week record of blood pressure **After 3 months:** Monthly record of blood pressure **Long-term high-dose therapy:** Close monitoring for lymphoproliferative disorders
Laboratory	Serum creatinine (2–3 measures and the average value is taken as baseline level) Blood urea Urinalysis Complete blood count ESR Liver function test Serum lipid profile Serum electrolytes (potassium and magnesium) Serum uric acid Mantoux test Hepatitis B and C serology	**Initial 3 months:** *Every-other-week* Serum creatinine Blood urea Complete blood count *Monthly* Complete blood count Liver function test Serum lipid profile Serum electrolytes (potassium and magnesium) Serum uric acid **After 3 months:** *Monthly* Serum creatinine Blood urea **Therapy > 1 year:** Serum creatinine monthly Glomerular filtration rate yearly **Patients on >3 mg/kg dosage or hepatic compromise:** CsA blood level

Indications

In the context of dermatological emergency, it is the first line of drug in psoriatic erythroderma. It may be used in erythroderma due to other causes like:
- Pityriasis rubra pilaris
- Reiter's disease
- Norwegian scabies.

In immunobullous disorders it may be used as an adjuvant drug.

Dose

Methotrexate is available as both oral and parenteral preparation. Oral tablets are available in various strengths (2.5 mg, 5 mg, 7.5 mg, 10 mg) and the injectable form may be administered through intramuscular, intravenous and subcutaneous routes. The drug is administered at a dosage of 2 to 3 mg/kg body weight, once in a week as single or 2 to 3 divided doses. In dermatological conditions, e.g. psoriasis, the maximum intravenous dose must be < 50 mg/week.

The oral dose is administered after feeding and folic acid supplementation (5 mg/day) is continued.

Adverse Effects

Adverse effects which may be encountered with administration of MTX in a patient with psoriatic erythroderma admitted in dermatological intensive care unit include:
- Acute onset mucositis and mucosal erosions involving oral (ulcerative stomatitis) and gastrointestinal tract.
- Gastric intolerance like anorexia, nausea, vomiting and diarrhea.
- Myelosuppression, causing individual cytopenia or pancytopenia.

In presence of any of these side effects, the drug has to be withdrawn temporarily, with cautious readministration.

Contraindications
Absolute Contraindications
- Pregnant and lactating patients
- Active infection, acute or chronic, like tuberculosis
- Patients with positive hepatitis B, C and HIV serology
- Advanced hepatic and renal disease.

Relative Contraindications
- Altered hepatic and renal function.

Patient Monitoring While on MTX Therapy
Baseline, Before Starting Treatment
- Thorough clinical examination to rule out active infection
- Complete hemogram and ESR
- Urinalysis
- Liver function test
- Renal function test
- Hepatitis B, C and HIV serology.

While the Patient is on Treatment
- Look for gum bleeding, epistaxis, hematuria or continued bleeding from venipuncture sites.
- Evidence of infection (upper respiratory tract/urinary tract infection/pyoderma).
- Complete blood count to be repeated on 7th day and thereafter at interval of every 1 to 2 weeks or with clinical evidence of cytopenias, e.g. active bleeding/infection. If total WBC count is < 3500/mm^3 and platelet count is < 100,000, the drug should be withheld temporarily.
- Liver function test (if serum transaminase levels are > 2 times the normal values, either the dosage has to be reduced or the drug is withdrawn temporarily.

Patient's response to methotrexate is monitored by estimating disease activity (PASI score to be done at baseline and thereafter every 1–2 weeks).

Drug Interactions
Important drugs to be avoided during MTX therapy are:
- Trimethoprim-sulfamethoxazole (enhanced risk of toxicity)
- NSAIDs (decrease renal excretion of MTX)
- Anticonvulsant; phenytoin (displacement from plasma protein, increased free MTX).

Methotrexate Toxicity
Management of methotrexate toxicity has been discussed in detail in chapter 9 under rescue therapy.

CYCLOPHOSPHAMIDE

It is a cytotoxic drug (alkylating agent) commonly used for various malignant conditions. It has been used by rheumatologists and dermatologists also, as an immunomodulator.

Indications
In the context of dermatological emergency, cyclophosphamide may be used in following conditions:
- As adjuvant therapy, in immunobullous disorders like pemphigus and pemphigoid
- Erythroderma due to connective tissue disorder, e.g. dermatomyositis
- Erythroderma due to mycosis fungoides (advanced stage disease)
- It may constitute a component of chemotherapy in patients presenting with erythroderma due to other lymphoproliferative disorders.

Dose

Cyclophosphamide is available as oral (25 mg, 50 mg tablet) and intravenous injections. Usual dose is 2 to 3 mg/kg. In patients with pemphigus it constitutes a component of dexamethasone-cyclophosphamide pulse (DCP) therapy and is administered as monthly once bolus intravenous injection (reconstituted drug administered as slow IV injection) on first day of pulse; on completion of pulse, 50 mg of oral tablet is continued till next cycle.

Adverse Effects

- Leukopenia/thrombocytopenia/anemia
- Nausea, vomiting and diarrhoea
- Bladder toxicity giving rise to dysuria, hematuria and hemorrhagic cystitis.

Contraindications

Absolute Contraindications

- Pregnant and lactating patients

Relative Contraindications

- Altered hepatic and renal function
- Active infection.

Patient Monitoring While on Cyclophosphamide Therapy

Baseline, before starting treatment:
- Clinical examination to rule out active infection
- Complete blood count
- Urine microscopy.

While the patient is on treatment:
- Complete blood count, initially weekly, thereafter monthly. If total WBC count is < 4000/mm^3 and platelet count < 100,000, the drug should be withheld temporarily.
- If there is RBC in urine, provided other causes are ruled out, the drug should be withheld temporarily.

Management of Cyclophosphamide Toxicity

- As a preventive measure for bladder toxicity oral dose is administered in morning and patient is instructed to drink plenty of oral fluid and void urine frequently. In patients receiving intravenous dose, an extra amount (500 ml 5% dextrose) of intravenous fluid may be administered if patient is too sick to drink water by himself.
- Management of hemorrhagic cystitis has been discussed in chapter 9.

VINCRISTINE

Vincristine has been used in Kassabach-Merritt phenomenon as an effective therapy to counter platelet destruction. It is thought to bind to the sequestered platelets.

Recommended Dose

Administered at a dose of 1 to 1.5 mg/m^2/week by slow intravenous transfusion. Most cases will show a response by 4 weeks with an average 12 weeks of treatment.

Outcome

This treatment appears to have a rapidly beneficial effect on the coagulopathy. Tumor shrinkage can be expected over a period of months.

In conclusion, dermatologists working in DICU must be conversant with the use of basic drugs used as life saver in critically ill patients. In addition, they should also remain updated regarding recent guidelines for use of various medications used for dermatological illnesses, like cyclosporine, methotrexate, etc. This is helpful in taking appropriate decision in a critically ill patient. Knowledge regarding adverse effects of drugs and drug-interactions help to manage patients with multisystem involvement.

SUGGESTED FURTHER READING

1. Bennett PN, Brown MJ. Adrenergic mechanisms and drugs. In: Bennett PN, Brown MJ, editors. Clinical pharmacology, 9th edition. Edinburgh: Churchill Livingstone; 2003.p-447-59.
2. Breathnach SM, Smith CH, Chalmers RJG, Hay RJ. Systemic therapy. In:Burns T, Breathnach S, Cox N, Griffiths C, editors. Rook's textbook of dermatology, 8th edition. Oxford: Wiley-Blackwell; 2010.p-74.1-74.54.
3. Brown AF. Anaphylactic shock: mechanisms and treatment. J Acad Emerg Med 1995;12:89–100.
4. Lee CS, Koo JYM. Cyclosporine. In: Wolverton SE, editor. Comprehensive dermatologic drug therapy, 2nd edition. Philadephia: Elsevier Saunders; 2007.p-219-37.
5. MacFie J. Nutrition and fluid therapy. In: Williams NS, Bulstrode CJK, O'Connell PR, editors. Bailey & Love's short practice of surgery, 25th edition. London:Hodder Arnold; 2008.p-222-33.
6. Manno M. Medications. In: Dieckmann RA, Fiser DH, Selbst SM, editors. Illustrated Textbook of Pediatric Emergency and Critical Care Procedures. St. Louis, Missouri: Mosby-Year Book; 1997.p-292-4.
7. Menter A, Korman NJ, Elmets CA, Feldman SR, Gelfand JM, Gordon KB, et al. Guidelines of care in the management of psoriasis and psoriatic arthritis. Section 4: Guidelines of care in the management and treatment of psoriasis with traditional systemic agents. J Am Acad Dermatol 2009;61:451-85.

8. Moss C, Shahidullah H. Naevi and other developmental defects. In:Burns T, Breathnach S, Cox N, Griffiths C, editors. Rook's textbook of dermatology, 8th edition. Oxford:Wiley-Blackwell; 2010.p-18.1-18.108.
9. Stralen DV, Perkin RM. Oxygen delivery. In: Dieckmann RA, Fiser DH, Selbst SM, editors. Illustrated Textbook of Pediatric Emergency and Critical Care Procedures. St. Louis, Missouri: Mosby-Year Book; 1997.p-125-32.
10. Thomas K, Ruetter A, Luger TA. Intravenous immunoglobulin therapy. In: Wolverton SE, editor. Comprehensive dermatologic drug therapy, 2nd edition. Philadephia: Elsevier Saunders; 2007.p-459-69.
11. Wolverton SE. Systemic Corticosteroids. In: Wolverton SE, editor. Comprehensive dermatologic drug therapy, 2nd edition. Philadephia: Elsevier Saunders; 2007.p-127-61.
12. Wyatt R. Anaphylaxis. How to recognize, treat and prevent potentially fatal attacks. Postgrad Med 1996;100:87–90.
13. Yu Z, Lennon VA. Mechanism of intravenous immune globulin therapy in antibiody-mediated autoimmune disease. N Engl J Med 1999;340: 227–8.

Rescue Therapy in Dermatology

Arun C Inamadar, Murlidhar Rajagopalan

- Cyclosporine as rescue therapy
- Infliximab as rescue therapy
- Corticosteroid as rescue therapy
- Rescue therapy in methotrexate toxicity
- Rescue therapy in dapsone induced methemoglobinemia
- Rescue therapy in cyclophosphamide induced bladder toxicity
- Other indications of rescue therapy in dermatology

INTRODUCTION

Rescue therapy refers to nonsurgical medical treatment in life-threatening situations. Most physicians do not link rescue therapy to dermatology. However, rescue therapy in dermatology is useful in acute skin conditions or in chronic skin conditions like unstable psoriasis, which flares up suddenly. This is an exercise of risk stratification at diagnosis followed by intensive primary treatment in high-risk patients. This might effectively suppress inflammation and outcome may be better with reduced morbidity and mortality. Another facet where rescue therapy is used frequently in dermatology is during an unwanted effect of a drug threatening the patient's life. Rescue can also be implemented to prevent fatal complications during standard treatment. These aspects will be discussed briefly here.

Indications

Treatment of recalcitrant clinical conditions with "quick fix" agents:

- Cyclosporine in psoriasis and atopic dermatitis for managing flares.
- Infliximab in generalized pustular psoriasis (GPP)/Kawasaki disease.
- Steroid in Kawasaki disease.

Management of dreadful adverse effects of drugs:
- Antidotes in methotrexate toxicity.
- Methylene blue and other agents in dapsone induced methemoglobinemia.

Prevention of serious adverse effects of drugs:
- MESNA in cyclophosphomide induced bladder toxicity

Management of emergent infections in compromised hosts.

The "quick fix" agent is the drug that works rapidly, well-tolerated at high dose, and typically induces complete clearing. This therapy works better till the availability of another therapeutic agent to replace the 'quick fix' effectively. The best example is the use of cyclosporine in clearing phase of 'sequential therapy' of psoriasis. Rescue therapies for IVIg-resistant Kawasaki disease include methylprednisolone pulse or other steroid regimens, as well as infliximab, a tumor necrosis factor-α (TNF-α) antagonist. However, every rescue therapy in dermatology is not just a quick fix drug.

CYCLOSPORINE AS RESCUE THERAPY

Psoriasis

In psoriasis that has failed to respond to many other treatment modalities, cyclosporine works as a *'rescue therapy'*. This drug can also be used for acute pustular flares in psoriasis (**Figures 9.1A and B**). A maximum dermatological dose of 5 mg/kg daily is administered as two doses. As soon as the critical period is over, the dose of cyclosphorine A (CsA) should be decreased by 1 mg/kg/day every other week, till the minimum effective dose for maintenance therapy is achieved for the patient. It is always advisable to taper the dose of CsA gradually while an alternative therapy is

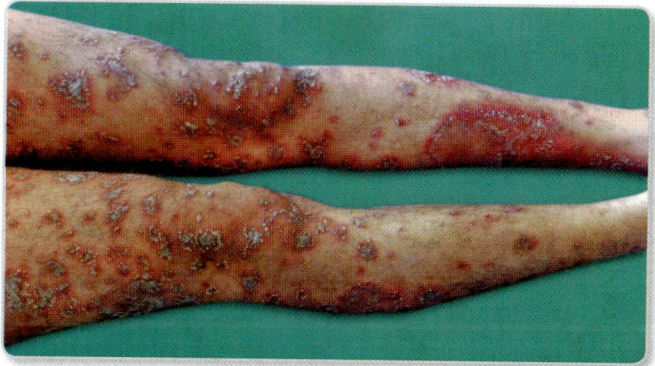

Figure 9.1A: Acute generalized pustular psoriasis

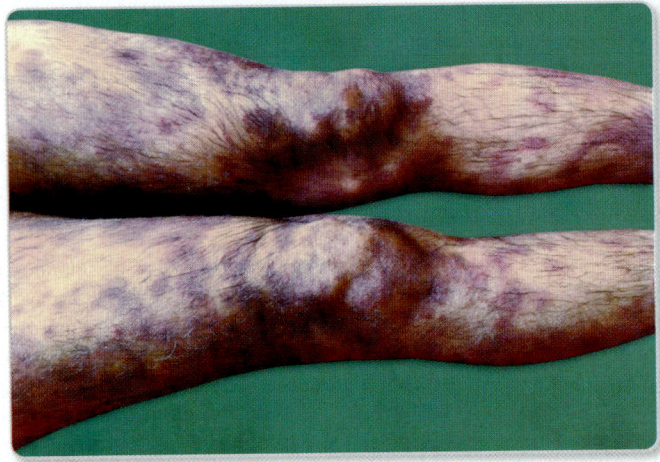

Figure 9.1B: Acute generalized pustular psoriasis following 2 weeks of treatment with cyclosporine

added. In some reports doses up to 10 mg/kg/day was required to induce a remission, before cyclosporine could be tapered.

Atopic Dermatitis

Atopic dermatitis (AD) is a classical dermatological illness where rescue therapy is essential during an acute flare. In many patients with chronic and mildly disabling disease the dermatologists may be able to manage the condition with emollients, topical steroids when needed, and tacrolimus or pimecrolimus used for long period. Some patients may need azathioprine for disease remission. Many children may need a brief course of systemic steroids.

A 'flare of AD' is defined as an episode requiring escalation of treatment or seeking additional medical advice. Consideration should also be given to totally controlled weeks and well-controlled weeks to assess overall disease activity in these patients. Thus, in a patient with AD who is resistant to standard therapy and still left with persistent, severe itching and flare of skin lesions, a rescue therapy is needed. A short course of cyclosporine, given at 3 mg/kg/day for three to four weeks is sufficient in most cases. Intravenous immunoglobulin (IVIg) may also be used to achieve control.

■ INFLIXIMAB AS RESCUE THERAPY

Generalized Pustular Psoriasis

TNF-α antagonists including infliximab have been used with success in treating recalcitrant cases of GPP of von Zumbusch. It is an unstable, inflammatory form of psoriasis, with the hallmark of neutrophilic infiltration in cutaneous as well as extracutaneous lesions. GPP is often recalcitrant, making treatment difficult. During a severe flare of GPP in a Chinese patient, a single dose of infliximab resulted in rapid clearing of cutaneous lesions, together with resolution of liver function abnormalities which was likely to be secondary to neutrophilic cholangitis. Subsequent maintenance therapy with acitretin resulted in remission of pustular disease for 7 months. Efficacy of single-dose infliximab for both cutaneous lesions and systemic hepatic involvement in generalized pustular psoriasis merits the role of infliximab as rescue therapy in GPP. Such single dose approach is also feasible economically in resource poor countries. In suitable patients infliximab is the preferred drug to treat GPP. Erythrodermic psoriasis is also another condition where the acute crisis in a patient may be managed with a biological like infliximab.

Kawasaki Disease

Current research has shown that TNF-α plays a role in inflammation in acute and refractory Kawasaki disease. Elevations in TNF-α receptors have been seen in patients with Kawasaki disease, with the highest levels occurring in those who develop coronary artery aneurysms after IVIg therapy. TNF-α antagonism with infliximab has shown potential as a *rescue therapy* for patients with persistent Kawasaki disease.

CORTICOSTEROID AS RESCUE THERAPY

Kawasaki Disease

Standard initial treatment for Kawasaki disease is a single dose of IVIg/2 gm/kg + aspirin 80–100 mg/kg/day. Patients with Kawasaki disease are deemed refractory or persistent cases, if the fever continues >36 hours after initial IVIg therapy. The role of steroid treatment in Kawasaki disease is controversial. Steroids have been used either as initial therapy or as rescue therapy after treatment failure with IVIg and aspirin. If more than two IVIg infusions are found to be ineffective, IV pulse methylprednisolone at 30 mg/kg over 2 to 3 hours, once a day for 1 to 3 days, should be administered.

In a recent study, combination treatment with intravenous immunoglobulin and prednisolone had a significant advantage as compared to intravenous immunoglobulin alone for prevention of coronary artery abnormalities in patients with severe Kawasaki disease. There was reduced need of additional rescue treatment, and more rapid resolution of fever and inflammatory markers in these patients.

RESCUE THERAPY IN METHOTREXATE TOXICITY

Methotrexate (MTX) is a chemotherapeutic drug that is structurally similar to folic acid. Methotrexate inhibits dihydrofolate reductase, an enzyme that reduces folic acid to tetrahydrofolic acid. Methotrexate is used in the treatment of a various dermatological conditions.

Methotrexate toxicity may develop due to increased patient susceptibility during treatment, excessive parenteral dose, therapeutic error by the patient (e.g. taking MTX orally daily instead of weekly dose), or intentional drug overdosage.

Primary route of elimination of MTX is renal. Patients with existing renal disease or with a potential for impaired renal function (e.g. those taking nephrotoxic drugs) are at increased risk of developing MTX toxicity. In addition, precipitation of MTX or its relatively insoluble metabolites in the renal tubules can cause acute renal failure and tubular necrosis, further impairing excretion. Persistently elevated serum concentration of MTX leads to hematological abnormalities, such as myelosuppression, and nonhematological effects like, stomatitis/mucositis and diarrhea, dermatitis, and hepatotoxicity.

Clinical manifestations of toxicity include nausea, vomiting, diarrhea, mucositis, stomatitis, esophagitis, elevated hepatic enzymes, renal failure, rash, myelosuppression (leukopenia, pancytopenia, and thrombocytopenia), acute lung injury, tachycardia, hypotension, and neurologic dysfunction. Toxic effects may occur in hours or days to weeks after MTX administration or during overdosage.

The management of MTX induced toxicity is as follows:
- General measure
- Antidotes : leucovorin, thymidine and glucarpidase
- Hemodialysis and hemoperfusion.

General Measures

Administration of activated charcoal is advocated in oral overdose of MTX. Adequate hydration and urinary alkalinization with sodium bicarbonate will prevent the renal failure. Intravenous fluids should be administered to reverse any volume depletion and to induce brisk diuresis (>60 mL/hour); this is critical to maximize MTX elimination. Since urinary precipitation of MTX is enhanced by aciduria, intravenous sodium bicarbonate is routinely given along with aggressive hydration to maximize urinary solubility. At pH 7.5 MTX is 10 times more soluble than at pH 5.5.

Antidotes

Leucovorin (folinic acid) is the reduced and active form of folic acid. It selectively rescues normal cells from the toxic effects caused by inhibition of the production of reduced folate by MTX. The recommended dosage in most cases is 100 mg/m^2 IV, every 3 to 6 hours until the plasma MTX level is < 0.01µmol/L or for ≥ 3 days, if MTX levels are not available.

Folinic acid rescue also controls the gastrointestinal side effects of MTX toxicity. In most patients, this is not required if dose schedules are adhered to and routine folic acid supplementation is given when the patient is on MTX. Routine folic acid supplementation does not interfere with the therapeutic benefits of methotrexate. This is one example of 'long-term rescue therapy' in dermatology, anticipating the potential side effects of a drug.

Thymidine rescues cells from the cytotoxic effects of MTX. Its use is investigational and is given only along with other therapies.

Glucarpidase (carboxypeptidase) is an antidote that has been used recently for MTX toxicity in combination with leucovorin. It converts MTX to an inactive form and rapidly lowers blood level of MTX. It is given as a single bolus of 50 units/kg IV over 5 minutes. Leucovorin should be continued for 48 hours after glucarpidase administration. It is mainly used if there is MTX toxicity due to intrathecal overdosage.

RESCUE THERAPY IN DAPSONE INDUCED METHEMOGLOBINEMIA

Dapsone is used in a number of dermatological conditions other than leprosy. One of the adverse effects is methemoglobinemia. Acute methemoglobinemia constitutes a medical emergency and if severe, may result in significant mortality inspite of treatment.

Clinical symptoms vary according to the methemoglobin concentration. Cyanosis develops at methemoglobin level >1.5 g/dL. Acidosis, bradycardia, seizures, coma, arrhythmia and death may occur at methemoglobin level > 7.5 g/dL. Direct observation of blood while withdrawing may reveal that it has attained a chocolate brown color.

Treatment

Dapsone should be withdrawn immediately. Diluted methylene blue (MB), 1% sterile aqueous solution is administered as slow IV injection over 5 minutes. The recommended dosage schedule is as follows:
- Infants: 2 mg/kg.
- Older children: 1.5 mg/kg.
- Adults: 1 mg/kg.

The drug is available as an ampoule of 1% solution containing 10 mg/ml. MB powder can be reconstituted into a 1% solution and sterilized for IV use. Rapid relief is observed. If there is persistent cyanosis, dose can be repeated after an interval of 1 hour, till the maximum dose of 7 mg/kg over 24 hours.

If MB therapy is ineffective and life-threatening shock is imminent, exchange transfusion should be started. Additional therapy with activated charcoal is useful in dapsone induced methemoglobinemia. Other therapeutic modalities in use are ascorbic acid (if MB is contraindicated), N-acetylcysteine and hyperbaric oxygen.

RESCUE THERAPY IN CYCLOPHOSPHAMIDE INDUCED BLADDER TOXICITY

Mesna (sodium 2-mercaptoethane sulfonate) is a drug used to reduce the undesired side effects of certain chemotherapeutic drugs. It is referred to as a "chemoprotectant". Cyclophosphamide is one of the components of dexamethasone-cyclophosphamide-pulse (DCP) therapy, used in the management of pemphigus vulgaris. Cyclophosphamide is also indicated in various dermatological disorders as immunomodulator/adjuvant therapy or as steroid sparing agent. Well-known complication of cyclophosphamide is bladder toxicity presenting as hemorrhagic cystitis. The toxicity is probably due to the acrolein metabolite of cyclophosphamide. Cyclophosphamide should be discontinued once hematuria is noted. Mesna is used for the prevention of high dose cyclophosphamide-induced hemorrhagic cystitis. Mesna helps to detoxify these metabolites like acrolein by replacement of its sulfhydryl group with the vinyl group. It also increases urinary excretion of cysteine.

Mesna is not normally required with relatively low dose cyclophosphamide like that used in DCP therapy where 500 mg is typically used. However, when higher immunoablative doses are used which can produce side effects and even cytopenia, it is required as a routine. At present it is administered intravenously; an oral form is being investigated. Mesna (dosage equivalent to 60–160% w/w of the daily cyclophosphamide dosage), is administered by IV injection (in 3-5 divided doses daily) or by continuous IV infusion.

OTHER INDICATIONS OF RESCUE THERAPY IN DERMATOLOGY

Immunoablative High Dose Cyclophosphamide

The use of immunoablative IV cyclophosphamide (50 mg/kg/day for 4 days) without stem cell rescue has been described in patients with refractory autoimmune diseases such as paraneoplastic pemphigus, systemic lupus erythematosus, and aplastic anemia. Dermatologists occasionally encounter pemphigus patients who are refractory to all forms of therapy and have extensive disease. In such situation high dose cyclophosphamide can be used as rescue therapy, keeping in mind to give mesna to rescue the patient from cyclophosphamide toxicity. In this form of rescue therapy for pemphigus, cyclophosphamide is used in doses of 50 mg/kg/day for three to four days. Sepsis and thrombocytopenia should be anticipated and treated immediately. This form of therapy may result in a cure of refractory pemphigus. Stem cell rescue is not given here.

Prevention of Herpes Simplex Mucositis in Bone Marrow Transplant or Stem Cell Transplant Patients

In patients receiving bone marrow transplant (BMT) who are seropositive for herpes simplex virus (HSV)-1, the incidence of reactivation of HSV ranges from 65 to 90%. This may provide a portal of entry for other oral pathogens into the blood stream. Acyclovir may be effective against this reactivation when administered prophylactically. However, acyclovir has a low bioavailability and frequent dosage schedule. Valacyclovir is a prodrug of acyclovir and well absorbed in the gut. This provides for convenient twice or thrice oral daily dose. Valacyclovir can be given prophylactically at a dose of 500 mg twice daily until the resolution of neutropenia.

In conclusion, a general overview of rescue therapy in dermatology has been presented herewith. As the subject expands and the effects of newer drugs are better understood, we can expect newer indications and a better understanding of rescue therapy. The definition of rescue therapy in the context of dermatology may itself change in the future.

SUGGESTED FURTHER READING

1. Burns JC, Mason WH, Hauger SB, Janai H, Bastian JF, Julie D., et al. Infliximab treatment for refractory Kawasaki syndrome. J Pediatr 2005; 146:662–7.
2. Chandran NS, Chong WS. A dramatic response to a single dose of infliximab as rescue therapy in acute generalized pustular psoriasis of von Zumbusch associated with a neutrophilic cholangitis. Australas J Dermatol 2010;51:29–31.
3. Kobayashi T, Saji T, Otani T, Takeuchi K, Nakamura T, Arakawa H. Efficacy of immunoglobulin plus prednisolone for prevention of coronary artery abnormalities in severe Kawasaki disease (RAISE study): a randomised, open-label, blinded-endpoints trial. Lancet 2012;379:1613–20.

chapter 10

Dermatological Drug Therapy in Challenging Clinical Scenarios

Ragunatha S

- Dermatological drug therapy in patients with renal impairment
- Dermatological drug therapy in patients with hepatic impairment

INTRODUCTION

It is easier to take decision in the management of otherwise healthy patients with primary cutaneous disorders. With advances in the health care facilities, dermatologists are likely to see more number of patients with multiple comorbidities. These include renal impairment, hepatic impairment, immunodeficiency states, etc. Dermatological disease in a patient with these comorbidities presents a challenging clinical scenario. While treating such patients, several important issues need to be considered.

As many pathophysiological changes occur in different organ systems in these patients, there is a possibility of change in the course of both the diseases. In addition, pharmacokinetic and pharmacodynamic properties of the drugs are altered depending upon underlying organ involvement. Multiple medications administered to the patients increase the risk of toxicity and drug interactions. In such a situation, conventional treatment may lead to inadequate therapeutic response or adverse drug reactions. Therefore, the management strategy and the drug regimen which are used in patients without comorbidities need to be modified.

The clinical trials evaluating the efficacy and safety of the drugs used in dermatological diseases usually include healthy individuals without comorbidities. The influence of dermatological condition and associated comorbidity on each other is also not completely understood due to lack of studies. Kidney and liver are the two major organs responsible for elimination of drugs and their metabolites from the body. In this chapter more common and important clinical scenarios such as dermatological drug therapy in renal and hepatic impairment has been discussed.

DERMATOLOGICAL DRUG THERAPY IN PATIENTS WITH RENAL IMPAIRMENT

Chronic kidney disease (CKD) is fast becoming a global health problem. Diabetes and hypertension along with increased life expectancy are the leading causes of CKD worldwide. Hence, dermatologists are likely to see more number of patients with concomitant renal impairment. Chronic kidney disease is characterized by progressive deterioration of kidney function. The decline in the excretory function of the kidneys results in altered pharmacokinetics of the drugs and subsequent toxicity or change in therapeutic response. Therefore, appropriate dosage adjustment for the drugs eliminated by kidneys is essential. Drug dosage adjustment depends on:
- Renal drug clearance
- Degree of renal impairment
- Practical considerations.

Thorough understanding of these factors is important in avoiding dosing errors in patients with renal impairment.

Renal Drug Clearance

Three processes, in combination, are responsible for renal elimination of a drug. These are:
- *Glomerular filtration:* It is a low clearance process where only unbound drug in plasma is excreted. The drugs bound to large molecules like albumin and alpha-acid glycoprotein are not filtered through glomeruli.
- *Active tubular secretion:* Here, drugs with high protein binding are actively secreted in proximal convoluted tubules (PCT) and excreted. The PCT cells are equipped with various transport proteins which mediate excretion of number of drugs and their metabolites according to their chemical nature.
- *Tubular reabsorption:* Here, the drugs are reabsorbed into the circulation through passive diffusion. Lipophilic drugs have low renal clearance because of their extensive tubular reabsorption.

Pharmacokinetic Alterations in Renal Impairment

In addition to altered elimination, renal impairment also affects bioavailability, protein binding, distribution and hepatic metabolism of various drugs in the following ways:
- Uremia decreases the gastrointestinal (GI) absorption of the drugs. Increased gastric pH, gastroparesis and associated GI symptoms contribute significantly to the decreased absorption and bioavailability of drugs.
- CKD is associated with hypoalbuminemia leading to increased free concentration of acidic drugs (e.g. beta-lactum antibiotics) which bind to albumin.

- The volume of distribution of drugs varies with change in extracellular fluid (ECF) volume. The hydrophilic and highly protein bound drugs tend to have large volume of distribution (Vd) in presence of edema and ascites (increased ECF volume) leading to decreased serum concentration. Muscle wasting and increased adipose tissue decreases volume of distribution leading to increased serum concentration of the hydrophilic drugs (e.g. penicillin).
- Hepatic metabolism is impaired in CKD. In general, phase I reactions like hydrolysis and reduction, and phase II reactions like acetylation, methylation, glucorunidation and sulfation are slowed down resulting in increased serum drug concentrations.

Dose Adjustment of Drugs in Renal Impairment

In view of variations in pharmacokinetics of drugs, experts have warned against the oversimplification of complexities of renal drug clearance in patients with CKD and solely relying on drug information references which give only general guidelines for dose adjustment. Therefore, to avoid dosing errors in CKD, a stepwise approach is recommended which provides a framework for dose adjustment. These guidelines and approach are adapted or modified according to individual patient's specific situation. Usually the dosage adjustment is not required for drugs whose non-renal elimination is >70% (**Table 10.1**).

Table 10.1: Dermatological drugs whose dosage adjustment is not required in renal failure

Sl. no	Class of drugs	Drugs
1	Antibacterials	Amoxycillin, Azithromycin, Ceftriaxone, Cefuroxime (oral), Chloramphenicol, Clindamycin, Dicloxacillin, Doxycycline, Linezolid, Metronidazole, Minocycline, Moxifloxacin, Nafcillin, Rifabutin, Spectromycin, Tigecycline
2	Antifungals	Itraconazole, Ketoconazole, Griseofulvin, Posaconazole, Voriconazole, Anidulafungin, Miconazole
3	Antivirals	Nevirapine, Efavirenz, Indinavir, Abacavir, Saquinavir, Ritonavir, Atazanavir
4	Analgesics	Diclofenac, Ibuprofen, Indomethacin
5	Immunosuppressants	Hydrocortisone, Prednisone, Prednisolone, Triamcinolone, Methyl prednisolone, Betamethasone, Dexamethasone, Tacrolimus
6	Antidepressants	Amitryptiline, Nortryptiline, Imipramine, Doxepine, Fluoxetine
7	Others	Carbamazepine, Phenytoin, Clofazimine, Diazepam, Propranolol, Ondansetron, Omeprazole, Etanercept, Infliximab, Penicillamine

Initial Patient Assessment

The patient is evaluated in detail about:
- Nature of the renal impairment; acute or chronic, determined based on rapidity with which it had developed. The type of renal injury is identified, glomerular, tubular, vascular or interstitial. Compared to acute renal failure, patients with CKD are at higher risk of dosing errors, drug interactions and multiple organ involvement.
- History of previous drug reactions.
- Current medication list; usually, patients with CKD take multiple drugs prescribed for various associated ailments. Therefore, it is important to identify potential nephrotoxic drugs (**Table 10.2**) and rule out possibility of major drug interactions.
- Underlying organ involvement; CKD is associated with multi-organ involvement which may alter the pharmacodynamic effects of the drugs. Due care should be taken while choosing a drug which may cause toxicity of already damaged organ.
- Anthropometric measurements; anthropometric measurements, like height and weight are recorded for dosage calculation.

Table 10.2: Commonly used dermatological drugs causing nephrotoxocity

Sl. no	Type of nephrotoxicity	Drugs
1	Prerenal injury	Amphotericin B, Cyclosporine, Nonsteroidal anti-inflammatory drugs (NSAIDs), Tacrolimus
2	Acute tubular necrosis	Aminoglycosides, Amphotericin B, Immunoglobulin, Outdated Tetracycline
3	Allergic interstitial nephritis	Acetaminophen, Acyclovir, Aminoglycosides, Amphotericin B, Carbamazepine, Cephalosporins, Ciprofloxacin, Cyclosporine, Indinavir, NSAIDs, Omeprazole, Penicillamine, Penicillins, Phenytoin, Ranitidine, Rifampin, Sulfonamides, Vancomycin
4	Glomerular injury	NSAIDs, Penicillamine
5	Thrombotic microangiopathy	Cyclosporine, Tacrolimus
6	Intratubular obstruction	Acyclovir, Gancyclovir, Indinavir, Methotrexate, Sulfonamides
7	Chronic renal failure	Chronic analgesic abuse, Cyclosporine, Tacrolimus

Assessment of Renal Impairment

Glomerular filtration rate (GFR) is considered as a reliable and surrogate index of renal function. Extent of decrease in GFR indicates the degree of renal impairment. Hence, GFR is routinely used to assess the overall kidney function. Based on GFR, CKD is categorized into five stages:

- Stage I (Normal, GFR >90 ml/min/1.73m^2)
- Stage II (mild, 60–89 ml/min/1.73m^2)
- Stage III (moderate, 30–59 ml/min/1.73m^2)
- Stage IV (severe, 15–29 ml/min/1.73m^2)
- Stage V (end stage renal disease, <15 ml/min/1.73m^2).

The first two stages are asymptomatic with normal kidney function. Dosage adjustment is required for last three stages of CKD. For routine evaluation of renal function, GFR is determined by calculating creatinine clearance.

Among many equations, Cockcroft-Gault equation is commonly used to calculate creatinine clearance:

> Creatinine clearance (Cl_{cr}) in males = (140 − Age) × Weight ÷ 72 × serum creatinine
> Creatinine clearance in females = [(140 − Age) × Weight ÷ 72 × serum creatinine] × 0.85
> (Cl_{cr} is expressed in ml/min, weight in kg, age in years and serum creatinine in mg/dl).

Selection of Loading Dose

Adjustment in loading dose is necessary for drugs (e.g. aminoglycosides) with large Vd and narrow therapeutic index. In the presence of volume depletion loading dose of such drugs is decreased by 25%. The loading dose is increased if there is extracellular volume excess. If rapid therapeutic level has to be achieved, the administration of loading dose is necessary for all drugs. The loading dose is calculated by using the following formula:

> Loading dose = Vd × IBW × Cp
> (Vd = volume of distribution in liters/kg, IBW = ideal body weight in kg, Cp = desired plasma concentration in mg/liter).

Selection of Maintenance Dose

Administration of correct maintenance dose is essential to achieve a steady blood concentration of drug, and reduction of chances of subtherapeutic dose or toxicity. In patients with renal failure, it is accomplished by:

- Dosage reduction method; dose administered at each interval is reduced keeping the interval between doses unchanged.

- Interval extension method; only time interval between individual doses is increased.
- Combination of both.

The extent of dosage reduction or interval extension depends upon the degree of renal impairment (**Tables 10.3** and **10.4**). Interval extension method is suitable for drugs with long half-life and wide therapeutic range. The risk of drug toxicity is high in dosage reduction method. Hence, sometimes combination of both methods is necessary to provide optimum therapeutic response with minimal toxicity.

Monitoring Outcomes

Though, many drug information references are available for dosage adjustment in renal failure, these give different recommendations. Therefore, as mentioned above, references should be used as general guidelines because these do not ensure therapeutic efficacy and prevention of toxicity. Whenever available, drug level monitoring is advised to individualize the therapy. Clinical monitoring is also important because toxicity can occur at therapeutic range in the presence of metabolic derangement or multiple organ involvement.

Drug Dosing in Dialysis

Various procedures designed for dialysis remove the drugs and their active metabolites in addition to toxic metabolic wastes, necessitating dosage adjustment. In patients with renal failure on hemodialysis, dosage adjustment is advised as for patients with GFR <10 ml/min (**Table 10.4**). If patient is on continuous renal replacement therapy, dosage adjustment as for patients with GFR 10-50 ml/min (**Table 10.3**) is recommended. Smaller size (<500 daltons), more hydrophilic and less protein bound drugs undergo higher clearance during dialysis. For the drugs significantly removed by dialysis, administration is scheduled after the dialysis session to avoid drug loss.

Drug Dosing in Acute Renal Failure

As in CKD, both pharmacokinetic and pharmacodynamic properties of the drugs are altered in acute renal failure (ARF) also. However, there is no reliable method to estimate GFR in patients with ARF as, following acute renal injury it takes time for serum creatinine to be elevated. There are no guidelines or pharmacokinetic studies available for dosage adjustment in patients with ARF. Therefore, regular monitoring of drug levels and toxicity is essential.

DERMATOLOGICAL DRUG THERAPY IN PATIENTS WITH HEPATIC IMPAIRMENT

Liver plays an important role in absorption, distribution and elimination of majority of the drugs and their active or inactive metabolites. Liver is a major

Table 10.3: Dosage adjustment for drugs if GFR is 10–50 ml/min

Drugs	Method	Dosage	Drugs	Method	Dosage
Paracetamol	I	q 6 h	Lincomycin	I	q 6–12 h
Acyclovir	D, I	5 mg/kg q 12–24 h	Lomefloxacin	D	50–100%
Amikacin	D, I	3–4 mg/kg q 24 h	Methotrexate	D	50%
Amphotericin B	I	q 24 h	Mycophenolate	D	50–100%
Ampicillin	I	250 mg–2g q 6 h	Nelfnavir		No data
Azathioprine	D	75–100%	Nicotinic acid		50%
Cefepime	D, I	50–100% q 24 h	Norfloxacin	I	q 12–24 h
Cefixime	D	75–100%	Ofloxacin	D	50%
Cefotaxime	I	q 6–12 h	Penicillamine		Avoid
Ceftazidime	I	1–2g q 24 h	Penicillin G	D	75%
Cefuroxime (IV)	I	q 8–12 h	Pentoxyfylline	I	q 12–24 h
Cephalexin	I	250–500 mg q 8–12 h	Pentamidine	I	q 24 h
Ciprofloxacin	D	50–100%	Piperacillin	I	q 6–12 h
Clarithromycin	D	75%	Pregabalin	D	50% q 8–12 h
Cyclophosphamide	D	75–100%	Ribavirin		Avoid
Didanosine	D	33–50%	Rifampin	D	50–100%
Emtricitabine	I	q 48–72 h	Spironolactone	D	50%
Ethambutol	I	q 24–36 h	Stavudine	D, I	50% q 12–24 h

Contd...

Contd...

Drugs	Method	Dosage	Drugs	Method	Dosage
Famciclovir	I	q 12–24 h	Streptomycin	I	q 24–72 h
Fexofenadine	I	q 12–24 h	Sulfamethoxazole	I	q 18 h
Gabapentin	D,I	300 mg q 12–24 h	Tazobactum	D	75%
Ganciclovir	I	1.25–2.5 mg/kg q 24 h	Ticarcillin	I	50–75 mg/kg q 8 h
Gentamicin	D,I	2–3 mg/kg/day	Tramadol	D,I	50–100 mg q 8 h
Hydroxyurea	D	50%	Trimethoprim	I	q 12 h
Hydroxyzine	D	50%	Vancomycin	D,I	1 g q 24–96 h
Infliximab		No data	Zalcitabine	I	q 12 h
Lamivudine	D,I	50–150 mg q 24 h	Zidovudine	D,I	100% q 8 h
Levofloxacin	D	50%			

Note: D, Dosage reduction method; h, hour; I, Interval extension method; IV, Intravenous; q, every

Table 10.4: Dosage adjustment for drugs if CFR is <10 ml/min

Drugs	Method	Dosage	Drugs	Method	Dosage
Paracetamol	I	q 8h	Hydroxyzine	D	50%
Acyclovir	D, I	2.5–5 mg/kg q 24 h	Infliximab		No data
Amikacin	D, I	2 mg/kg q 24–48 h	Isoniazid	D	75–100%
Amphotericin B (liquid)	I	q 24 h	Lamivudine	D, I	25–50 mg q 24 h
Ampicillin	I	250 mg–1 g q 6 h	Levofloxacin	D	25–50%
Azathioprine	D	50–100%	Lincomycin	I	q 12–24 h
Cefadroxil	I	q 24 h	Lomefloxacin	D	50%
Cefepime	D, I	25–50% q 24 h	Methotrexate		Avoid
Cefixime	D	50%	Mycophenolate	D	50–100%
Cefotaxime	I	1 g q 8–12 h	Nicotinic acid	D	25%
Cefpodoxime	I	100–200 mg q 24–48 h	Norfloxacin	I	q 24 h
Ceftazidime	I	0.5–1 g q 48 h	Ofloxacin	D	25%
Cefuroxime (IV)	I	750 mg q12 h	Penicillamine		Avoid
Cephalexin	I	250–500 mg q 12–24 h	Penicillin G	D	20–50%
Cetirizine	D	50%	Pentoxyfylline	I	q 24 h
Chloroquine	D	50%	Pentamidine	I	q 24–36 h
Chlorpheniramine	D	75–100%	Piperacillin	I	q 12 h
Ciprofloxacin	D	50%	Pregabalin	D, I	25% q 24 h

Contd...

Contd...

Drugs	Method	Dosage	Drugs	Method	Dosage
Clarithromycin	D	50–75%	Pyrazinamide	D	50–100%
Colchicine	D	50%	Ranitidine	D	50%
Cyclophosphamide	D	50–75%	Ribavirin		Avoid
Dapsone	D	50%	Rifampin	D	50–100%
Didanosine	D	25%	Spironolactone		Avoid
Emtricitabine	I	q 96 h	Stavudine	D or I	50% or q 24 h
Erythromycin	D	50–75%	Streptomycin	I	q 72–96 h
Ethambutol	I	q 48 h	Sulfamethoxazole	I	q 24 h
Famciclovir	D, I	50% q 24–48 h	Tazobactum	D	50%
Fexofenadine	I	q 24 h	Tetracycline	D	50%
Fluconazole	D	50%	Ticarcillin	I	50–75 mg/kg q 12 h
Gabapentin	D, I	300 mg q 48 h	Tramadol	D, I	50 mg q 8 h
Ganciclovir	I	1.25 mg/kg q 24 h	Trimethoprim	I	q 24 h
Gentamicin	D, I	2 mg/kg q 48–72 h	Vancomycin	D, I	1g q 4–7 days
Iloprost	D	50%	Zalcitabine	I	q 24 h
Hydroxyurea	D	20%	Zidovudine	D, I	50% q 8 h

Note: D, Dosage reduction method; h, hour; I, Interval extension method; IV, Intravenous; q, every

site of drug metabolism mediated by a diverse group of drug metabolizing enzymes. Hence, any change in liver function may lead to accumulation of drugs and their metabolites resulting in toxicity. To prevent drug induced liver injury and other adverse reactions, dosage adjustment is necessary in patients with hepatic impairment.

Hepatic Drug Clearance

Majority of the drugs which enter human body are lipophilic in nature. These drugs are metabolized by liver into hydrophilic molecules which are then excreted through urine and/or bile. The drugs taken orally undergo first metabolic transformation in the intestinal epithelial cells which contributes significantly to the progressive elimination of the drug. However, the total body clearance of the drug mostly depends on hepatic and/or renal elimination.

The three primary determinants of hepatic drug clearance are:
- Hepatic blood flow
- Protein binding of drugs
- Metabolism and biliary excretion of the drugs by enzyme activity.

Based on the efficiency of liver in removal of drugs from circulation, the drugs are categorized as having high, low or intermediate extraction ratio (**Table 10.5**).

Table 10.5: Classification of drugs according to hepatic extraction (%)

High extraction drugs (%) • Doxepin (74) • Zidovudine (85) **Intermediate extraction drugs (%)** • Amitryptiline (65) • Clarithromycin (40) • Erythromycin (37) • Nortryptiline (37) • Ondansetron (60) • Paracetamol (31) **Low extraction drugs (%)** • Acyclovir (4) • Amoxycillin (5) • Amphotericin B (2) • Ampicillin (3) • Carbamazepine (7) • Cefotaxime (15) • Ceftriaxone (2) • Cetirizine (2) • Chloroquine (25) • Ciprofloxacin (15)	• Clindamycin (15) • Cyclosporin (20) • Dexamethasone (20) • Diazepam (2) • Dicloxacillin (5) • Doxycycline (2) • Ethambutol (10) • Famciclovir (10) • Indomethacin (9) • Isoniazid (14) • Lincomycin (4) • Methotrexate (1) • Metronidazole (3) • Ofloxacin (5) • Penicillin G (9) • Piperacillin (4) • Prednisolone (9) • Ranitidine (2) • Rifampicin (17) • Vancomycin (1) • Cotrimoxazole (1) • Streptomycin (1)

Note: Estimation of hepatic extraction ratio of drugs is indirect and may therefore be inaccurate

Dosage Adjustment in Patients with Liver Disease

Any liver disease which significantly affects the above three factors, results in altered pharmacokinetics of drugs necessitating dosage adjustment. Liver diseases other than cirrhosis result in mild alterations in pharmacokinetics of drugs. Therefore, dosage adjustment is recommended mainly for patients with cirrhosis and cholestasis.

Unlike in renal impairment where measurement of creatinine clearance is used for dosage adjustment, there is no such marker available in hepatic impairment, the measurement of which may guide drug therapy. However, Child-Pugh classification has been used to categorize the patients according to the severity of liver function impairment. The classification is based on five clinical and laboratory variables (**Table 10.6**):

- Serum bilirubin
- Serum albumin
- Prothrombin time
- Grade of encephalopathy
- Ascites.

Though the classification indicates degree of hepatic impairment, it does not correlate with the ability of the liver to metabolize individual drugs. Therefore, the extraction ratio of the drugs is considered for dosage adjustment.

Certain factors may increase the risk of hepatotoxicity induced by drugs. These include:

- Concomitant alcohol intake
- Age > 60 years
- Daily dose of drug > 50 mg
- Drugs with significant hepatic metabolism (>80%).

These factors should be evaluated in patients with liver disease before drug therapy. As far as possible, hepatotoxic drugs, especially those which may result in fatal outcome (**Table 10.7**) are avoided in patients with hepatic impairment.

Table 10.6: Child-Pugh classification

Clinical/biochemical indicator	Score		
	1	2	3
Serum bilirubin (mg/dL)	<2	2–3	>3
Serum albumin (g/dL)	>3.5	2.8–3.5	<2.8
Prothrombin time (s >control)	<4	4–6	>6
Encephalopathy (grade)	None	1 or 2	3 or 4
Ascites	Absent	Slight	Moderate

Class A (mild) = 5–6 points, Class B (moderate)= 7–9 points, Class C (severe)= 10–15 points

Table 10.7: Dermatological drugs causing acute hepatic failure

Sl. no	Class of drugs	Drugs
1	Antibacterials	Amoxycillin/Clavulanic acid, Azithromycin, Cefadroxil, Cefepime, Ciprofloxacin, Clarithromycin, Co-trimoxazole, Dapsone, Dicloxacillin, Doxycycline, Erythromycin, Ethambutol, Isoniazid, Levofloxacin, Norfloxacin, Piperacillin, Rifampicin
2	Antifungals	Itraconazole, Ketoconazole, Terbinafin
3	Antivirals	Abacavir, Didanosine, Lamivudine, Nelfinavir, Stavudine
4	Analgesics	Paracetamol, Diclofenac, Indomethacin, Nimesulide,
5	Others	Carbamazepin, Fluoxetine, Omeprazole, Sulfasalazine

Dosage Adjustment for High Extraction Drugs

The elimination of high extraction drugs mainly depends on hepatic blood flow. Patients with alcoholic cirrhosis often show decreased parenchymal blood flow compared to other forms of cirrhosis and irrespective of the etiology, parenchymal blood flow decreases later in the disease. A firm liver on palpation, small cirrhotic liver and decompensated state indicates severely reduced hepatic blood flow. Therefore, liver cirrhosis significantly increases the bioavailability of orally administered drugs. To avoid drug toxicity, both initial and maintenance doses of high extraction drugs have to be reduced. However, the extent of reduction cannot be determined because the accurate estimation of total hepatic blood flow and portal-systemic shunt is not possible. For drugs administered intravenously, a normal initial dose and reduction in maintenance dose is advised. The following equation can be used to calculate reduced initial and first maintenance dose:

$$\text{Reduced dose} = \text{Normal dose} \times \text{Bioavailability} \div 100$$

Where normal dose is the starting dose in a patient without liver disease, and bioavailability is derived from healthy individuals. The maintenance dose is adjusted based on desired therapeutic response and toxicity of the drug used.

Dosage Adjustment for Low Extraction Drugs with Low Binding to Albumin (<90%)

Bioavailability of these drugs is not significantly affected in hepatic impairment. The hepatic clearance of these drugs mainly depends on metabolic capacity and protein binding. The inter-individual variability of enzyme activity in cirrhosis makes it difficult to give accurate guidelines for dosage adjustment. Various studies have investigated dosage adjustment in hepatic impairment based on Child-Pugh classification. The recommendations for certain group of drugs from these studies are available for patients with class A or class B. The Child-Pugh class C patients have not been included in the studies because of ethical issues. The drugs for which no studies are available, it is recommended to administer a maintenance dose of 50% of normal dose in patients belonging to class A and 25% of normal dose in patients belonging to class B. The dose is further adjusted according to the pharmacological effects and toxicity. In Child-Pugh class C patients only drugs which are not metabolized in liver and/or whose safety has been demonstrated in clinical trials are recommended.

Dosage Adjustment for Low Extraction Drugs with High Binding to Albumin (>90%)

The free fraction of high protein binding drugs is significantly increased even with slight decrease in albumin levels. This free fraction is rapidly metabolized by the liver. Hence, in patients with liver cirrhosis with associated hypoalbuminemia, the total plasma concentration is decreased when their free concentration is in normal range. To avoid toxicity by overdosage, free drug concentration is determined to guide the therapy.

Dosage Adjustment for Intermediate Extraction Drugs

In general, hepatic clearance of these drugs is reduced. The treatment should be started with low range of normal dose and the maintenance dose is adjusted as for low extraction drugs based on Child-Pugh classification.

Renal Clearance of Drugs in Patients with Liver Disease

The patients with advanced hepatic disease have reduced renal plasma flow and GFR. The estimation of GFR from serum creatinine in patients with cirrhosis is inaccurate because of impaired synthesis of creatinine by the liver. Therefore, the drugs with predominant renal elimination should be administered with caution.

In conclusion, selection of appropriate drugs is critical in the management of dermatological patients with renal or hepatic impairment. Though, there are general guidelines for dosage adjustment in these comorbid conditions, the drug is administered cautiously and titrated individually till the desired pharmacological effects are achieved or at appearance of toxicity. Due to lack of data on pharmacokinetic properties and dosage adjustment in renal or hepatic impairment, guidelines have been given to pharmaceutical companies to carry out detailed pharmacokinetic study of newer drug in the setting of impaired renal and hepatic function, and to include patients with these disorders in the clinical trial through careful selection.

SUGGESTED FURTHER READING

1. Bircher J, Sommer W. Drug treatment in patients with liver disease. In: Bircher J, Benhamou J-P, McIntyre N, Rizzetto M, Rodes J, editors. Oxford Textbook of Clinical Hepatology, 2nd edition. Oxford: Oxford Medical Publication; 1999.p-1983-94.
2. Bjornsson E. Review article: drug induced liver injury in practice. Aliment Pharmacol Ther 2010;32:3–13.
3. Delco F, Tchambaz L, Schlienger R, Drewe J, Krahenbuhl S. Dose adjustment in patients with liver disease. Drug Safety 2005;28:529–45.
4. Hassan Y, Al-Ramahi RJ, Aziz NA, Ghazali R. Drug use and dosing in chronic kidney disease. Ann Acad Med Singapore 2009;38:1095–1103.
5. McIntyre CW, Shaw S, Eldehni MT. Prescribing drugs in kidney disease. In: Tall MW, Chertow GM, Marsden PA, Skorecki K, Yu ASL, Brenner BM, editors. Brenner and Rector's The Kidney, 9th edition. Philadelphia: Elsevier Saunders; 2012.p-2258-89.
6. Suzuki A, Andrade RJ, Bjornsson E, Lucena MI, Lee WM, Yuen NA, et al. Drugs associated with hepatotoxicity and their reporting frequency of liver adverse events in VigiBaseTM. Drug Safety 2010;33:503–22.
7. Swan SK, Bennett WM. Drug dosing guidelines in patients with renal failure. West J Med 1992;156:633–8.
8. Verbeeck RK, Musuamba FT. Pharmacokinetics and dosage adjustment in patients with renal dysfunction. Eur J Clin Pharmacol 2009;65:757–73.
9. Verbeeck RK. Pharmacokinetics and dosage adjustment in patients with hepatic dysfunction. Eur J Clin Pharmacol 2008;64:1147–61.

chapter 11

Drugs in Pregnancy and Lactation

Laxmi Nair

- Physiological changes in pregnancy and their effect on pharmacokinetics
- Drug dosing in pregnancy
- Prenatal development and relationship with maternal drug intake
- Pharmacokinetics of drugs ingested by the mother in the fetus
- Drug categorization during pregnancy
- Drug prescription in lactating women
- Monitoring and management principles

INTRODUCTION

Drug prescription for a pregnant woman is often a dilemma for physicians. Some of the pertinent questions before taking a decision are:

- Is the drug safe?
- Will it have any adverse effect on the growing fetus?
- Is the drug or its metabolites secreted in the breast milk?

Awareness of the potential dangers of medication during pregnancy began when the teratogenic effects of thalidomide were first recognized. Prior to this, there was a general belief among clinicians and patients that developing embryo and fetus is protected *in utero* by the "placental barrier." The placental barrier was believed to insulate the fetus from substances ingested by the mother.

A pregnant woman is as susceptible to illness as any other person and many pregnant women do require treatment for herself as well as for the well-being of the fetus. The data available on the effect of drugs on the fetus and the breast-fed babies is inadequate and quite conflicting. This is one of the least-developed areas of clinical pharmacology and drug research. As a result, many women are either refused treatment or experience potentially harmful delay in receiving medication. On the other hand, some apparently safe drugs are prescribed despite evidence of possible teratogenicity.

Only few medications have been tested for safety and efficacy during pregnancy and lactation. In many cases, the safety of a drug cannot be determined until it has been widely used. There is a potential for adverse effects on the mother and fetus though evidence based human studies are lacking. The risk of major congenital malformations in general population is 2%, hence a drug need not necessarily be blamed for a malformation but it is always preferable to avoid litigation for prescribing a drug that is blamed to be responsible for the problem.

If the pregnant woman has other comorbid conditions there is potential for drug interactions too. Newer drugs are being introduced at a fast pace and it is often difficult to remain up to date; yet physicians need to be well informed about the drugs used in daily practice and their effects on pregnancy and lactation. It is a challenge for clinicians to keep abreast of the latest recommendations and best practice guidelines for treating pregnant and lactating women. Safety of a given drug may again vary trimester-wise, some drugs are safe during one stage of pregnancy but not in another. Knowledge regarding safety profile of commonly prescribed drugs enables a doctor to prescribe with confidence.

One way to find out the effect of drugs on the unborn baby is by the use of 'pregnancy registry'. A pregnancy registry is a study that enrolls women when they have been taking a drug during pregnancy. Babies born to these women are compared to the babies of women who have not taken any drug during pregnancy. A large data is needed over a period of time before conclusions can be drawn.

The populations at risk are:
- Women on medication just prior to conception.
- Women who conceive while on medication.
- Pregnant women who need to take medication.

PHYSIOLOGICAL CHANGES IN PREGNANCY AND THEIR EFFECT ON PHARMACOKINETICS

Physiological changes during pregnancy have the potential to alter the absorption, distribution, metabolism and elimination of drugs used by the pregnant women. These changes include:

- Plasma volume expansion.
- Increase in extracellular fluid space and total body water.
- Decreased plasma albumin concentration.
- A compensated respiratory alkalosis.
- Increased cardiac output with changes in regional blood flow.
- Increased renal blood flow associated with increased glomerular filtration.
- Changes in hepatic drug metabolizing enzymes.
- Changes in gastrointestinal function.
- Ventilatory changes.

These changes begin in early gestation and become most pronounced in the third trimester of pregnancy. Maternal physiological changes may also take place during intrapartum period. Some of these changes are normalized within 24 hours of delivery. Others may persist till around 12 weeks postpartum. The effects of various physiological changes during pregnancy on drug metabolism have been presented briefly in **Table 11.1**.

Table 11.1: Physiological changes in pregnancy and related effects on drug administration

System	Physiological change during pregnancy	Effect on drug administration
Cardiovascular	↑Blood volume (40–50%) ↑Cardiac output (50%) ↑Heart rate	
Renal	↑Glomerular filtration rate (50%)	Faster renal clearance of certain drugs
Gastrointestinal	Vomiting due to morning sickness ↓ gastric acid ↑ gastric emptying time ↓ gastrointestinal motility	↓ drug absorption ↑ oral bioavailability of slowly absorbed drugs ↓ peak plasma concentration of rapidly absorbed drugs
Hepatic	Induction of hepatic enzymes Estrogen/progesterone: – Induces cytochrome P-450 system – Competitive inhibition of certain enzymes Estrogen induced cholestasis	↓ in level of drugs eliminated by hepatic metabolism ↑ metabolism and elimination of certain drugs ↓ elimination of certain drugs ↓ clearance of drugs (rifampicin)
Respiratory	Changes in ventilation	↓ absoption of inhaled drugs
Metabolic changes	↓ albumin ↑ total body water (approx. 8 liters)	↑ concentration of unbound acidic drugs, which undergo hepatic metabolism and overall drug concentration remains unaltered ↓ peak serum concentration of certain drugs

DRUG DOSING IN PREGNANCY

In view of the paucity of studies, presently it is not possible to formulate therapeutic guidelines in pregnancy for the safe use of drugs and dosing schedules for individual drugs. In order to design evidence-based guidelines for drug dosing in pregnancy, high-quality pharmacokinetic studies of adequate sample size which incorporate a nonpregnant control group are required. On current evidence, dose requirements are likely to be higher for drugs with increased clearance during pregnancy. Dose titration for protein-bound drugs should be based on monitoring of free drug concentration.

PRENATAL DEVELOPMENT AND RELATIONSHIP WITH MATERNAL DRUG INTAKE

The process of prenatal development occurs in three main stages. The first two weeks after conception is the germinal stage; the third through the eighth week is the embryonic period; and the time from the ninth week until birth is the fetal period. Cell division continues at a rapid rate and develops into a blastocyst. The blastocyst is made up of three layers:

- The *ectoderm* (skin and nervous system)
- The *endoderm* (digestive and respiratory systems)
- The *mesoderm* (muscle and skeletal systems).

During the germinal stage any insult to the developing organs will have an all or none effect, either death and abortion or survival of the embryo by rapid multiplication of the still totipotential cells to replace those that have been lost.

It is during the 18 to 55 days after conception that the basic steps in organogenesis occur. The embryo begins to divide into three layers each of which will become an important body system. Approximately 22 days after conception, the neural tube forms and later develops into the central nervous system including the spinal cord and brain. It is during the embryonic period that major congenital malformations are more likely to occur following intake of teratogenic drugs. The earlier the insult occurs the greater is the likelihood of effect.

Around the fourth week, the head begins to form followed by facial structures. The earliest activity starts in the cardiovascular system, heart is formed and starts to pulsate. During the fifth week, limb buds appear.

By eight weeks, the embryo has all of the basic organs and body parts except the sex organs. Once cell differentiation is mostly complete, the embryo enters fetal stage. The early body systems and structures established in the embryonic stage continue to develop. During the fetal stage drugs may lead to defects in growth and functional loss rather than gross structural abnormalities.

PHARMACOKINETICS OF DRUGS INGESTED BY THE MOTHER IN THE FETUS

Most drugs cross the placenta and there is little information about their effect during first trimester. Drug transfer occurs mainly via diffusion across the placenta, favoring the movement of lipophilic agents, and the rate-limiting step is the placental blood flow. Following are some of the general principles of pharmacokinetics of various drugs in mother and the fetus during pregnancy:

- Protein-bound drugs, and drugs with large molecular weight (e.g., heparin and insulin), do not cross the placenta.
- Both the immature fetal liver and the placenta can metabolize drugs. At 8 weeks postconception, immature phase I and phase II metabolism can occur in the fetus. However, fetal hepatic enzyme activity is low, and this coupled with the fact that 50% of the fetal circulation from the umbilical vein bypasses the fetal liver contributes to the problem of fetal drug accumulation.
- Elimination of drugs from the fetus is by diffusion back into the maternal compartment. Because most drug metabolites are polar, this favors accumulation of metabolites within the fetus.
- As the kidney develops, more drug metabolites are excreted into the amniotic fluid. This may theoretically lead to prolonged exposure of the fetus by way of skin contact or by ingestion of amniotic fluid.
- Drugs may also be accumulated within the fetus by `ion trapping'. The basis for this is the slightly more acidic pH of the fetal plasma as compared to mother. Weak bases (nonionized, lipophilic drugs) diffuse across the placental barrier and become ionized in the more acidic fetal blood, leading to a net movement from the maternal to fetal system.

The drug effects depend on its dose and the stage of development of the fetus. It is not only the teratogenic potential of the drugs, dose and time of exposure to the drugs determines whether there is significant teratogenic risk or no risk at all. Following are some of the factors determining the risks related to maternal drug intake to the fetus:

- During the very early stage (within 20 days of fertilization), the fetus is highly resistant to birth defects.
- During 3rd and 8th weeks after fertilization (period of organogenesis), vulnerability to birth defects is most.
- Drugs taken beyond this period are unlikely to result in obvious birth defects, but may affect the growth and function of normally formed organs and tissues. The period of insult determines which structures are more susceptible to be affected.
- In late trimesters, exposure to a drug results into potential functional damage, referred to as fetotoxicity. These defects may be permanent but

subtle, e.g. nonsteroidal anti-inflammatory drugs may cause fetal renal dysfunction in the 2nd and 3rd trimesters and premature closure of the ductus arteriosus in the 3rd trimester.
- Drugs may affect the fetus indirectly by causing:
  - Placental vasoconstriction and thus reducing the supply of oxygen and nutrients.
  - Contraction of uterine muscles reducing blood supply to the baby.

These may lead to intrauterine growth retardation. Some drugs may result in early, delayed or even prolonged labor.

Gestational period at which various organs are at risk of developing malformations due to drug administration have been presented in **Table 11.2**.

DRUG CATEGORIZATION DURING PREGNANCY

Clinicians are guided by the US Food and Drug Administration (US FDA) categorization of drugs (based on risk) for advising medications during pregnancy.

The pregnancy category of a drug is an assessment of the risk of fetal injury if it is used in the mother during pregnancy. It does not include

Table 11.2: Risk of various organ involvements by drugs during pregnancy

Preorganogenesis (Initial 2 weeks)	Organs/body parts affected	Embryonic period (3–8 weeks) Major malformations	Fetal period (9 weeks—term) Minor malformations or functional defects
	Central nervous system	3rd week to early 6th week	6th week to term
	Heart	Mid 3rd week to late 6th week	End of 6th week to 8th week
	Ear	Early 4th week to early 9th week	9th to 12th week
	Eyes	Mid 4th week to mid 8th week	Late 8th week to term
No effect/abortion	Limb	Mid 4th week to 7th/early 8th week	8th to early 9th week
	Lips	Mid 5th week to early 6th week	Late 6th week
	Teeth	Mid 6th week to 8th week	9th to 20th week
	Palate	Late 6th week to early 9th week	Late 9th week
	External genitalia	Mid 7th week to 9th week	Late 9th week to term

any risks conferred by the drug or its metabolites that are present in breast milk. **Table 11.3** presents the US FDA definitions for the pregnancy categories. One characteristic of the US FDA definitions is that a relatively large amount of high quality data on a pharmaceutical product is required to categorize as 'A'; hence many drugs which can be considered as pregnancy category A in other countries are allocated to category C by the FDA. This system does not address the risk of not treating a disease versus the risks of the medication.

Other countries have different systems of pregnancy categorization of drugs, e.g. in Australia the subdivision of category B into B1, B2 and B3; in Germany the categories are designated as Gr1 to Gr11. Detailed discussion on these is beyond the scope of this chapter.

Following are some of the general rules regarding prescribing drugs in pregnancy:

- It is generally thought that drugs in FDA category A are always perfectly safe during pregnancy. However, an unforeseen problem may occur, though the risk of harm is very low.
- Category B drugs are often prescribed in pregnancy. These are considered safe, although there may be some risk of birth defects in animals and may

Table 11.3: Pregnancy category of drug prescription (US FDA)

Pregnancy category	Description
A	No demonstrable risk to the fetus in 1st trimester and no evidence of risk in later trimesters of pregnancy in well-controlled human studies
B	No demonstrable risk to the fetus in animal studies but there are no adequate and well-controlled human studies OR Animal studies have shown adverse effects, but adequate and well-controlled human studies have failed to demonstrate a risk to the fetus in any trimester
C	Animal studies have shown adverse effects, and there are no adequate and well-controlled human studies; however, potential benefits may allow use of the drug in pregnant women despite potential risks
D	Human fetal risk evidenced by adverse reaction data from investigational or marketing experience; however, potential benefits may warrant use of the drug in pregnant women despite potential risks
X	Demonstrable fetal abnormalities in animal models as well as in human studies AND/OR Positive evidence of human fetal risk evidenced by adverse reaction data from investigational or marketing experience, and the risks involved with use of the drug in pregnant women clearly outweighs potential benefits

or may not have been tested for safety in pregnant women. A category B drug is safer for human use than a category C drug.
- Category C drug should be avoided in pregnancy unless there is a clear need and no alternatives available from category A or B. Potential benefit may warrant the use of the drug despite the risk.
- Category D drugs should be avoided in pregnancy when possible, but are not absolutely contraindicated in pregnancy, unlike those in category X.

Despite the shortcomings, the system of pregnancy categorization is a guide to determine the potential risk of maternal drug administration to the fetus. A detailed list of pregnancy categorization of various drugs prescribed by dermatologists has been presented at the end of this chapter (**Appendix 1**). For a quick reference on the risk of drugs during pregnancy and lactation, following website may be visited; **www.safefetus.com**

DRUG PRESCRIPTION IN LACTATING WOMEN

Lactating women who are prescribed drugs for various ailments are always concerned about its effect on their babies. As most drugs are excreted into the milk by passive diffusion, the drug concentration in milk is directly proportional to maternal plasma concentration. The milk to plasma (M:P) ratio, which compares milk with maternal plasma drug concentrations, serves as an index of the extent of drug excretion in breast milk.

For most drugs the amount ingested by the infant through breast milk rarely attains therapeutic level. Nearly all drugs reach breast milk in doses < 1% of the maternal dose but only a few drugs pose a risk to the breastfed baby. Very few drugs are contraindicated during breastfeeding. As a general rule lactating women should take a drug only on absolute indications and for a minimum necessary period. It is preferable to avoid drugs with long half lives, sustained-release preparations, or drugs with high M:P ratio. Milk:Plasma ratio of ≥1 indicates that more of the drug is secreted into the milk.

While prescribing drugs in lactating women following general rules may be followed:

- The dose schedule may be altered in such a way that the least amount of it is secreted in breast milk (mother may take the medicine after a feeding, preferably after night feeding, rather than before nursing).
- The age and health status of the infant must be taken care of. Prematurity, low birth weight or illness put an infant at higher risk of drug effects. Exposure to drugs in breast milk should be avoided in such infants.
- In general, antineoplastic drugs, drugs of abuse, some anticonvulsants, ergot alkaloids, and radiopharmaceuticals should not be taken by lactating women.

There are very few studies on the effects of drugs taken by a mother on her breastfed infant. Evidence of harmful effects of a drug in a breastfed baby is based on case reports, clinical experience and anecdotal reports. Some of the dermatological drugs contraindicated during lactation have been listed in **Table 11.4**.

Table 11.4: Dermatological drugs contraindicated during lactation

Category X drugs	*Retinoids:* Etretinate, Isotretinoin, Acitretin, Tazarotene (topical) *Antineoplastic drugs:* Cyclophosphamide, Methotrexate, 5-Fluorouracil *Others:* Estrogens, Finasteride, Flutamide, Stanozolol, Thalidomide
Medications decreasing milk production	Bromocriptine, Diuretics

MONITORING AND MANAGEMENT PRINCIPLES

While treating a woman of childbearing age, it should be ascertained whether the patient is using contraception, planning a pregnancy, is pregnant, or is lactating, before treatment for a dermatologic illness is prescribed. A careful history of the recent dates of her periods and the menstrual cycle is important. If the patient is on contraceptive drug or device, the possible interaction with the prescribed drug, if any, should be ascertained, as failure of contraception is a risk to the patient. If patient is trying to conceive, she must be advised to inform the doctor as soon as she becomes pregnant. If the patient is pregnant and needs a drug that places her or the fetus at risk, the dermatologist should discuss this with her and the family, and document the discussion about the potential risk. In situations when there is a significant risk, the risk benefit ratio needs to be assessed and discussed with the patient, informed consent should be obtained and documented. If the patient is near term, dermatologic drugs that are contraindicated during the last two weeks should be taken note of.

Women who are on drugs for a chronic illness should be counseled before their pregnancy so as to increase the awareness of the risks of teratogenesis and how to reduce the chances of fetal malformation. They should also be told about the adverse effects of untreated illness on the fetus. Women who have taken a drug without knowing that they are pregnant also need to be counseled.

In conclusion, while treating pregnant women a delicate balance between possible harms and benefits to both the mother and fetus should be maintained. A drug should only be used if the benefit outweighs the risk. No drug should be used in pregnancy without a reasonable indication. Drug dosing may need to be changed in pregnancy because of the increased volume of distribution and increased renal and hepatic drug clearance. Newly introduced medications should preferably be avoided because many important drug toxicities in pregnancy have only been identified during post marketing surveillance.

■ SUGGESTED FURTHER READING

1. Acyclovir. In: Briggs GG, Freeman RK, Yaffe SL, editors. Drugs in pregnancy and lactation, 7th edition. Baltimore: Lippincott Williams and Wilkins; 2005. p-23–9.
2. Adalimumab. In: Briggs GG, Freeman RK, Yaffe SL, editors. Drugs in pregnancy and lactation, 7th edition. Baltimore: Lippincott Williams and Wilkins; 2005. p-29–30.
3. Adapalene. In: Briggs GG, Freeman RK, Yaffe SL, editors. Drugs in pregnancy and lactation, 7th edition. Baltimore: Lippincott Williams and Wilkins; 2005. p-30–31.
4. Adverse Drug Reactions Advisory Committee. Premature closure of the fetal ductus arteriosus after maternal use of non steroidal anti inflammatory drugs. Med J Aust 1998;164:444–51.
5. Altschuler DZ, Kenney LR. Pediculocide performance, profit, and the public health. Arch Dermatol 1986;122:259–61.
6. American Academy of Pediatrics Committee on Drugs. Transfer of drugs and other chemicals into human milk. Pediatrics 2001;108:776–89.
7. Aspirin. In: Briggs GG, Freeman RK, Yaffe SL, editors. Drugs in pregnancy and lactation, 7th edition. Baltimore: Lippincott Williams and Wilkins; 2005. p-105–13.
8. Azithromycin. In: Briggs GG, Freeman RK, Yaffe SL, editors. Drugs in pregnancy and lactation, 7th edition. Baltimore: Lippincott Williams and Wilkins; 2005. p-140–2.
9. Benzathine Penicillin. Available at: www.drugs.com/breastfeeding/benzathine-penicillin-g.html Accessed on 30th June, 2012.
10. Boubred F, Vendemmia M, Garcia-Meric P, Buffat C, Millet V, Simeoni U. Effects of maternally administered drugs on the fetal and neonatal kidney. Drugs Saf 2006;29:397–419.
11. Brent RL, Fawcett LB. Developmental toxicology, drugs and fetal teratogenesis. In: Reece EA, Hobbins JC, editors. Clinical Obstetrics: The Fetus and Mother, 3rd edition. Malden, MA: Blackwell Publishing Inc; 2007. p-217–35.
12. Buhimschi CS, Medications in pregnancy and lactation: part 1. Teratology. Obstet Gynecol 2009;113:166–188.
13. Buttar HS, Moffatt JH, Bura C. Pregnancy outcome in ketoconazole treated rats and mice. Teratology 1989;39:444.
14. Cefaclor, cephalexin, cephradine. In: Briggs GG, Freeman RK, Yaffe SL, editors. Drugs in pregnancy and lactation, 7th edition. Baltimore: Lippincott Williams and Wilkins; 2005. p-241–72.
15. Cleary BJ, Källén B. Early pregnancy azathioprine use and pregnancy outcomes. Birth Defects Res A Clin Mol Teratol 2009; 85: 647–54.
16. Clindamycin Topical Official FDA information, side effects and uses. Available at: www.drugs.com/pro/clindamycin-topical.html. Accessed on 30th June, 2012.
17. Cyclosporine. In: Briggs GG, Freeman RK, Yaffe SL, editors. Drugs in pregnancy and lactation, 7th edition. Baltimore: Lippincott Williams and Wilkins; 2005. p- 405–8.

18. Dapsone. In: Briggs GG, Freeman RK, Yaffe SL, editors. Drugs in pregnancy and lactation, 7th edition. Baltimore: Lippincott Williams and Wilkins; 2005. p- 424–7.
19. Dawes M, Chowienczyk PJ. Drugs in pregnancy. Pharmacokinetics in pregnancy. Best Pract Res Clin Obstet Gynaecol 2001;15:819–26. Available at: http://www.idealibrary.com Accessed on 30th June, 2012.
20. Doxepin. In: Briggs GG, Freeman RK, Yaffe SL, editors. Drugs in pregnancy and lactation, 7th edition. Baltimore: Lippincott Williams and Wilkins; 2005. p-513–6.
21. Einarson A, Bailey B, Jung G, Spizzirri D, Baillie M, Koren G. Prospective controlled study of hydroxyzine and cetirizine in pregnancy. Ann Allergy Asthma Immunol. 1997;78:183–6.
22. Etanercept. In: Briggs GG, Freeman RK, Yaffe SL, editors. Drugs in pregnancy and lactation, 7th edition. Baltimore: Lippincott Williams and Wilkins; 2005. p-596–8.
23. Famciclovir. In: Briggs GG, Freeman RK, Yaffe SL, editors. Drugs in pregnancy and lactation, 7th edition. Baltimore: Lippincott Williams and Wilkins; 2005. p-626–7.
24. Fexofenadine. In: Briggs GG, Freeman RK, Yaffe SL, editors. Drugs in pregnancy and lactation, 7th edition. Baltimore: Lippincott Williams and Wilkins; 2005. p-639–40.
25. Fluconazole. In: Briggs GG, Freeman RK, Yaffe SL, editors. Drugs in pregnancy and lactation, 7th edition. Baltimore: Lippincott Williams and Wilkins; 2005. p-648–53.
26. Food and Drug Administration. Federal Register. 1980;44:37434–67.
27. Fraser FC, Sajoo A. Teratogenic potential of corticosteroids in humans. Teratology 1995;51:45–6.
28. Frederiksen MC. Physiologic changes in pregnancy and their effect on drug disposition. Semin Perinatol 2001;25:120–123.
29. Gunnarskog JG, Källén AJB, Lindelöf BG, Sigurgeirsson B. Psoralen photochemotherapy (PUVA) and pregnancy. Arch Dermatol 1993;129:320–3.
30. Hanretty KP, Whittle MJ. Identifying abnormalities. In: Rubin P, editor. Prescribing in pregnancy, 2nd edition. London: BMJ Publishing Group; 1995. p- 8–21.
31. Honein MA, Paulozzi LJ, Himelright IM, Lee B, Cragan JD, Patterson I, et al. Infantile hypertrophic pyloric stenosis after pertussis prophylaxis with erythromycin: a case review and cohort study. Lancet 1999;354:2101–5.
32. Hydroxyzine. In: Briggs GG, Freeman RK, Yaffe SL, editors. Drugs in pregnancy and lactation, 7th edition. Baltimore: Lippincott Williams and Wilkins; 2005. p-794–7.
33. Imiquimod, topical. In: USP DI: drug information for the health care professional. Greenwood Village (CO): Thomson Micromedex; 2005. p- 1650–2.
34. Imiquimod. Available at: medscape.com/drug/aldara-zyclara-imiquimod-343508. Accessed on 30th June, 2012.
35. Infliximab. In: Briggs GG, Freeman RK, Yaffe SL, editors. Drugs in pregnancy and lactation, 7th edition. Baltimore: Lippincott Williams and Wilkins; 2005. p-832–4.
36. Itraconazole. In: Briggs GG, Freeman RK, Yaffe SL, editors. Drugs in pregnancy and lactation, 7th edition. Baltimore: Lippincott Williams and Wilkins; 2005. p. 869–71.

37. Kallen B. The teratogenicity of antirheumatic drugs- what is the evidence? Scand J Rheumatol 1998;27:119–24.
38. Ketoconazole. In: Briggs GG, Freeman RK, Yaffe SL, editors. Drugs in pregnancy and lactation, 7th edition. Baltimore: Lippincott Williams and Wilkins; 2005. p- 878–80.
39. Khir ASM, How J. Successful pregnancy after cyproheptadine treatment for Cushing's disease. Eur J Obstet Gynecol Reprod Biol 1981;13:343–7.
40. Leachman AA, Reed BR. The use of Drugs in Pregnancy and Lactation. Dermatol Clin 2006;24:168.
41. Li D-K, Liu L, Odouli R. Exposure to non-steroidal anti-inflammatory drugs during pregnancy and risk of miscarriage: population based cohort study. BMJ 2003;327:368–70.
42. Lipson AH, Collins F, Webster WS. Multiple congenital defects associated with maternal use of topical tretinoin. Lancet 1993;341:1352–3.
43. Loebstein R, Addis A, Ho E, Andreou R, Sage S, Donnenfeld AE, et al. Pregnancy outcome following gestational exposure to fluoroquinolones: a multicenter prospective controlled study. Antimicrob Agents Chemother 1998;42:1336–9.
44. Loebstein R, Lalkin A, Koren G. Pharmacokinetic changes during pregnancy and their clinical relevance. Clin Pharmacokinet 1997; 33:328–43.
45. Loratadine. In: Briggs GG, Freeman RK, Yaffe SL, editors. Drugs in pregnancy and lactation, 7th edition. Baltimore: Lippincott Williams and Wilkins; 2005. p- 940–2.
46. Medications during pregnancy and lactation. Available at: www.medscape.org/viewarticle/720225_2. Accessed on 30th June, 2012.
47. Meinking TL, Taplin D. Safety of permethrin vs. lindane for the treatment of scabies. Arch Dermatol 1996;132:959-62.
48. Menter A, Korman NJ, Elmets CA, Feldman SR, Gelfand JM, Gordon KB, et al. Guidelines of care for the management of psoriasis and psoriatic arthritis. Section 5. Guidelines of care for the treatment of psoriasis with phototherapy and photochemotherapy. J Am Acad Dermatol 2010;62:114–35.
49. Metneki J, Czeizel A. Griseofulvin teratology including two thoracopagus conjoined twins. Lancet 1987;1:1042.
50. Miconazole. In: Briggs GG, Freeman RK, Yaffe SL, editors. Drugs in pregnancy and lactation, 7th edition. Baltimore: Lippincott Williams and Wilkins; 2005. p-1076–7.
51. Morbidity and Mortality Weekly Report. Recommendations and Reports Sexually Transmitted Diseases Treatment Guidelines, 2010 December 7,2010/vol. 59/No. RR-12 p.18. Available at: http://www.cdc.gov/mmwr. Accessed on 30th June, 2012.
52. Morbidity and Mortality Weekly Report Recommendations and Reports Sexually Transmitted Diseases Treatment Guidelines, 2010 December 7,2010/vol. 59/No. RR-12 p. 74. Available at: http://www.cdc.gov/mmwr. Accessed on 30th June, 2012.
53. Morris LF, Harrod MJ, Menter MA, Silverman AK. Methotrexate and reproduction in men: case report and recommendations. J Am Acad Dermatol 1993; 29:913–6.
54. Mycophenolate. In: Briggs GG, Freeman RK, Yaffe SL, editors. Drugs in pregnancy and lactation, 7th edition. Baltimore: Lippincott Williams and Wilkins; 2005. p-1108–9.

55. Natekar A, Pupco A, Bozzo P, Koren G. Safety of azathioprine use during pregnancy. Available at: www.cfp.ca/content/57/12/1401. Accessed on 30th June, 2012.
56. Olopatadine. Available at: www.4nrx.com/allergies/allenil-olopatadine.html Accessed on 30th June, 2012.
57. Pacque M, Munoz B, Poetschke G, Foose J, Greene BM, Taylor HR. Pregnancy outcome after inadvertent ivermectin treatment during community-based distribution. Lancet1990;336:1486–9.
58. Park-*Wyl*lie L, Mazzotta P, Pastuszak A, Moretti ME, Beique L, Hunnisett L, et al. Birth defects after maternal exposure to corticosteroids: prospective cohort study and meta-analysis of epidemiological studies. Teratology 2000;62:385–92.
59. Parks AL. Antimalarial drugs, pregnancy and lactation. J Rheumatol 1993;2:S21–S23.
60. Pasternak B, Hviid A. Use of acyclovir, valacyclovir, and famciclovir in the first trimester of pregnancy and the risk of birth defects. JAMA 2010;304:859–66.
61. Powell RJ, Du Toit GL, Siddique N, Leech SC, Dixon TA, Clark AT, et al. British Society for Allergy and Clinical Immunology (BSACI). BSACI guidelines for the management of chronic urticaria and angio-oedema. Clin Exp Allergy 2007;37:631–50.
62. Rasmussen JE. Lindane, a prudent approach. Arch Dermatol 1987;123:1008–9.
63. Rayburn WF. Glucocorticoid therapy for rheumatic diseases: maternal, fetal, and breast-feeding considerations. Am J Reprod Immunol 1992;28:138–40.
64. Sau A, Clarke S, Bass J, Kaiser A, Marinaki A, Nelson-Piercy C. "Azathioprine and breastfeeding-is it safe?". BJOG 2007;114:498.
65. Schatz M. H1-antihistamines in pregnancy and lactation. Clin Allergy Immunol 2002;17:421–36.
66. Sugathan P, Riyaz N. Suppression of lactation by selenium disulphide. Int J Dermatol 1990; 29:232–3.
67. Tacrolimus. In: Briggs GG, Freeman RK, Yaffe SL, editors. Drugs in pregnancy and lactation, 7th edition. Baltimore: Lippincott Williams and Wilkins; 2005. p-1519–23.
68. Tagatz GE, Simmons RL. Pregnancy after renal transplantation. Ann Int Med 1975; 82: 113–4.
69. Terbinafine. In: Briggs GG, Freeman RK, Yaffe SL, editors. Drugs in pregnancy and lactation, 7th edition. Baltimore: Lippincott Williams and Wilkins; 2005. p-1537–8.
70. Thielitz A, Krautheim A, Gollnick H. Update in retinoid therapy of acne. Dermatol Ther 2006;19: 272–9.
71. Vitamin D. In: Briggs GG, Freeman RK, Yaffe SL, editors. Drugs in pregnancy and lactation, 7th edition. Baltimore: Lippincott Williams and Wilkins; 2005. p-1731–4.

Appendix

DERMATOLOGIC DRUGS DURING PREGNANCY AND LACTATION

Antihistamines

1st generation Category B

Chlorpheniramine, promethazine, dimenhydrinate, clemastine, mebhydroline, diphenhydramine
Controversy regarding use during lactation. Anticholinergic effects may inhibit lactation; risk of irritability/unusual excitement in infants. Mother should be advised to stop the drug if infant becomes jittery or stops feeding well.

2nd generation Category B

Cetirizine
In small prospective studies there is no increased risk to fetus. Can be used during lactation as only small amounts are found in breast milk.

Cyproheptadine
Safe during pregnancy.
Manufacturers' instruction is to avoid use during lactation.

Loratadine
Some adverse outcomes reported but no clear relationship found. Can be used during lactation, since only small amounts are found in breast milk.

Rupatadine
Excreted in animal milk. It is unknown whether it is excreted into human milk.

2nd generation Category C

Hydroxyzine
Limited safety data.

Doxepin Category (Systemic unrated, Topical B)

Olopatadine
No adequate and well-controlled studies in pregnant women. Lactation: Safety unknown

Ebastine: Pregnancy category not established.

3rd generation Category B

Levocetirizine
There are no data on excretion into human milk.

Category C

Desloratadine
No controlled study in human pregnancy and no data on the excretion into human milk.

Fexofenadine
Limited data. There are no controlled studies in human pregnancy and no data on excretion in human milk.

Antibacterial Agents

Category B

Azithromycin
No risk during pregnancy, to be used with caution during lactation.

Roxithromycin
Inadequate data from use in pregnant women. No teratogenic or fetotoxic effect in animal studies. It should not be used during pregnancy unless clearly indicated.
Lactation: Very small quantity of roxithromycin is excreted into maternal milk.

Erythromycin
Antibiotic of choice in pregnancy. No reported risk except for erythromycin estolate. To be used with caution during lactation.

Cephalosporins
No malformation identified in 2nd and 3rd trimester. To be used with caution during lactation.
A large surveillance study of Michigan Medicaid recipients (1985 to1992) observed a possible association between certain cephalosporins (cefaclor, cephalexin, ceftriaxone and cephadrine) and congenital malformations when taken in the first trimester.

Penicillins
Antibiotic of choice during pregnancy.
Beta-lactam penicillins: No increased risk of congenital anomalies.
Benzathine penicillin and procaine penicillin: Single maternal dose of benzathine penicillin G, 2.4 million units IM produce low levels in milk, not expected to cause adverse effects in breastfed infants.

Category C

Clarithromycin
In some animal studies low incidence of cardiovascular anomalies and cleft palate at doses close to human doses. No such reports in humans, but human data are limited.

Dapsone
Safe during pregnancy. Stopping treatment during the last month of pregnancy may minimize a theoretical risk of neonatal kernicterus.
Usually safe in lactation (American Academy of Pediatrics).

Fluoroquinolones
Possibility of joint abnormalities, seen only in animals. Possibility of congenital anomalies inconsistent. Should not be used as a first line drug.
Possibly compatible with lactation but manufacturers advice discontinuation of ciprofloxacin as potential adverse reactions may occur in infants.

Category D

Tetracycline
Use in early pregnancy is not associated with congenital anomalies. Occasionally, liver failure in the pregnant woman.
Slowed bone growth; use in second and third trimesters carries risk of permanent yellowing of the teeth and enamel hypoplasia.
Use controversial during lactation.

Contd...

Contd...

Minocycline
Structural similarity to tetracycline; so not advised during second and third trimester.

Doxycycline
Structural similarity to tetracycline; so not advised during second and third trimester.

Topical Acne Medications During Pregnancy

Category B

Erythromycin
Compatible with pregnancy and lactation.

Clindamycin
Safe in pregnancy and lactation. No adequate and well-controlled studies in pregnant women.
Should be used during pregnancy only if clearly needed.

Metronidazole
Topical use safe in pregnancy and lactation.

Azelaic acid
Minimally absorbed, risk in pregnancy unlikely. No risk in lactation.

Category C

Benzoyl peroxide absorbed in small amounts, not contraindicated in pregnancy or lactation.

Category C

Tretinoin: Not advised
Case reports of congenital malformations in infants whose mothers used tretinoin during the first trimester of pregnancy. No anomaly reported in infants of mothers treated during second and third trimesters.
Use during lactation is avoided as excretion via breast milk has not been studied and adverse reactions in infants have not been ruled out.
Rating should not be confused with X category isotretinoin.

Adapalene
Very low systemic absorption, potential benefit should be weighed against potential risk to infant during pregnancy.
It is doubtful that absorption might result in any risk during lactation.
Tazarotene is (category X) contraindicated in lactation.

Topical Antibiotics

Neomycin, bacitracin, mupirocin and polymyxin
Not associated with teratogenicity though large studies have not been conducted.

Silver sulphadiazine
In the third trimester, neonatal hemolysis and methemoglobinemia;
Increased risk of kernicterus in neonates appears to be unfounded. Kernicterus or hemorrhage in premature or glucose-6-phosphate dehydrogenase-deficient infants.

Antifungal Agents

The use of topical antifungals is considered safe in pregnancy because of negligible percutaneous absorption. Systemic therapy is not recommended in pregnancy and breastfeeding.

Topical

Category B
Clotrimazole Topical treatment of vaginitis in first trimester is associated with slightly increased risk of congenital defects in one study.
Ciclopirox olamine Not studied in humans. Not associated with risk in pregnancy.
Oxiconazole Not studied in humans. No risk in pregnancy.
Terbinafine No reports of risk in pregnancy. Probably safe in lactation.
Category C
Sertaconazole There is no data on the excretion of sertaconazole into human milk. Manufacturer recommends cautious administration in nursing women.
Eberconazole Not absorbed when topically applied.
Oxiconazole No adequate and well-controlled studies in pregnant women. Excreted in human milk. To be used with caution in lactating women.
Luliconazole No adequate well-controlled studies in pregnant women.
Miconazole: No association with congenital defects
Ketoconazole Topical form not studied in pregnant women. Probably safe in lactation.
Butaconazole Not studied in humans. No associated risk in pregnancy.
Selenium sulphide Not studied in humans or animals, hence risk to fetus is unknown. Suppression of lactation reported.
Butenafine No adequate well-controlled studies in pregnant women.
Amorolfine To be avoided in pregnancy and lactation though negligible fetal risk.

Oral Antifungal Agents

Category B

Terbinafine
Animal reproduction studies show low risk, but human pregnancy data are lacking. Potential toxicity during lactation.

Ketoconazole
Human and animal teratogenicity. To be avoided in first trimester.
Safe in lactating women.

Category C

Fluconazole
High doses during first two trimesters is associated with human malformations. Single dose use does not appear to be associated with increased risk to fetus.

Itraconazole
Available data pertaining to human use indicates no significant risk for major abnormalities but because of risk associated with use of fluconazole, a structurally related triazole antifungal, avoidance of itraconazole is suggested in the first trimester.

Griseofulvin: Unrated
Several reports implicate griseofulvin as a possible etiology for conjoined twins.
No risk in lactating women.

Antivirals in Pregnancy and Lactation

Category B
No significant association between first trimester exposure to acyclovir, valacyclovir and famciclovir and major birth defects.

Acyclovir
Safe during lactation.

Famciclovir
Used with caution during pregnancy. Contraindicated in lactation, as benign tumors may occur in rats.

Valacyclovir
Since valacyclovir is converted to acyclovir the effects during pregnancy and breastfeeding are same as acyclovir.

Biologic Agents

Category B

Adalimumab
No human studies have been conducted. No apparent evidence of embryotoxicity, teratogenicity or increased pregnancy loss.
Potential maternal benefits appear to be greater and probably outweigh the unknown fetal risk; treatment during the first trimester should be discussed with the patient.
No data available for use during lactation.

Etanercept
No evidence of adverse effects on humans, but the drug is very new.
Probably compatible with lactation.

Infliximab
Probably compatible with lactation. Manufacturer advises against breastfeeding during use.

Systemic Immunomodulatory and Antiproliferative Agents in Pregnancy and Lactation

Category X
Methotrexate Potent teratogenic; however, the risk may be very small. Women of childbearing age should use reliable birth control. Men should be counseled to possible reversible oligospermia and should avoid impregnating a woman while on methotrexate.
Category D
Azathioprine Risk of fetal affection is there and should not be prescribed in pregnant women without careful weighing of benefit versus the risks. There is no evidence of azathioprine resulting in congenital malformations, spontaneous abortions, or stillbirth, but increased risk of atrial or ventricular septal defects have been reported as compared to general population. Manufacturer advises not to breastfeed. Recent evidence suggest moderate safety of this drug and breastfeeding need not be withheld as immediate benefits may outweigh the risks.
Cyclophosphamide Contraindicated in pregnancy and lactation.
Category C
Cyclosporine Limited data shows use during pregnancy poses no risk to developing fetus. Use during lactation not recommended for risk of possible immunosuppression, effect on growth and association with carcinogenesis.
Mycophenolate mofetil Not recommended for use during pregnancy and lactation. Effective contraceptive must be used before, during, and six weeks after use.

Antimalarial Drugs

Chloroquine and hydroxychloroquine No congenital malformations on exposure during first trimester. Discontinuation of antimalarials should not be done during pregnancy Use in lactation is controversial; usually no adverse effect when taken during lactation.
Psoralens Probably mutagenic and teratogenic effect, but apparently PUVA treatment does not carry any significant risk for fetal abnormality. Lactation contraindicated for 24 hours after ingesting psoralen.

Corticosteroids in Pregnancy and Lactation

Category C

Systemic corticosteroids

Multiple studies on patients with steroid dependent systemic diseases showed no increased risk of congenital malformation. Use in high dosage during human pregnancy carries potential risk of placental insufficiency, low birth weight or stillbirth. Oral cleft may occur.

Risk of low birth weight exists with 10 mg/day dose administered any time during pregnancy.

Use during lactation is usually safe. Feeding may be delayed for 3–4 hours after the dose, to minimize exposure of the infant.

Topical corticosteroids

No significant risk to the fetus, if used during pregnancy. If large quantity is used over large body surface areas during pregnancy, there may be associated low birth weight.

Antiscabetics and Antipediculicides in Pregnancy and Lactation

Category B

Lindane

Use in pregnancy is controversial.

Lindane concentration in breast milk may increase for several days following topical application.

Alternative agent (e.g., permethrin) is recommended during pregnancy and lactation.

Malathion

This pediculicide is not associated with teratogenicity.

Permethrin

Lack of animal or human teratogenicity and absence of excretion into human milk make it a preferred treatment modality for scabies or head lice in pregnancy and lactation.

There are no data on the excretion of permethrin into human milk.

Category C

Ivermectin

Human teratogenicity and toxicity have not been observed. Avoidance during pregnancy is recommended.

Poorly excreted into breast milk. Amount ingested by the infant is small and not expected to cause any adverse effects.

Topical Immunomodulators in Pregnancy and Lactation

Imiquimod
Should not be used during pregnancy. Animal studies using toxic human doses have revealed fetal toxicities. Recommended in pregnancy when benefit outweighs risk.
Not shown to be secreted in human milk.

Pimecrolimus
No adverse outcome when used during pregnancy.
Manufacturer recommendation is not to use during lactation, but no evidence of secretion in breast milk.

Tacrolimus
No risk during pregnancy reported.
Manufacturer recommendation: use during lactation is contraindicated.

Miscellaneous Drugs

Category C

Calcipotriene
Topical use shows no fetal toxicity until maternal toxicity has been developed.
No risk identified with use during lactation.

Podophyllin and podofilox
Contraindicated during pregnancy.

Coal tar
No human studies have been conducted. No information is available on use during lactation.

Hydroquinone
This medication should be used during pregnancy only if clearly needed. To be used with caution in lactation; whether distributed in breast milk is not known.

Kojic acid
No data available.

Local Anesthetics

Category B

Lidocaine, Lidocaine + epinephrine and lidocaine + prilocaine
Not contraindicated in pregnancy and lactation in the doses used for small excisional biopsies.

Category C

Benzocaine
There are no controlled data in human pregnancy. There are no data on the excretion of benzocaine-trimethobenzamide into human milk.

Pramoxine
There are no controlled data in human pregnancy. No data on the excretion of pramoxine into human milk.

Analgesics

Category B
Acetaminophen
Analgesic of choice in pregnancy. Overdosage may result in hepato- or nephrotoxicity in infant or mother, may be used during lactation.
NSAIDs, like ibuprofen, naproxen, indomethacin and diclofenac are cyclo-oxygenase inhibitors. In the fetus and newborn, cyclooxygenase is a potent dilator of the ductus arteriosus and pulmonary resistance vessels. Its inhibition could potentially cause premature closure of these vessels. These drugs do not increase the risk of structural birth defects or other adverse effects. There is increased risk of spontaneous abortion in 1st trimester with use of NSAIDs. Use of NSAIDs beyond 30 weeks gestation is contraindicated because of their potential to cause premature closure of the fetal ductus arteriosus and persistent pulmonary hypertension. Ibuprofen, indomethacin, diclofenac, naproxen, piroxicam, ketorolac and tolmetin can be used during lactation.
Category C
Aspirin
Aspirin and other drugs containing salicylate are not recommended during pregnancy, especially during the last three months. Acetylsalicylate, may prolong the gestational period and may cause severe bleeding before and after delivery. To be avoided in last trimester as there is increased risk of cardiovascular and pulmonary dysfunction and oligohydramnios. Aspirin is excreted in human milk in small amounts and should be given to nursing mothers with caution. Depending upon maternal indication, decision should be made whether to discontinue nursing or the drug.

Index

A

Abdominal
    colic 37, 95
    CT scan 32
    girth 59
    pain 36, 40
Acetylation 216
Acid base balance and correction of electrolytes 183
    calcium chloride 183
    calcium gluconate 183
    sodium bicarbonate 183
Acneiform lesions 166
Activated partial thromboplastin time 193
Acute
    airway obstruction 167
    cutaneous drug reactions (ACDR) classifications of
        less severe ACDRs 166
        severe ACDRs 166
    generalized pustular psoriasis 20
    graft versus host disease 109
        clinical clues 110
        differential diagnosis 110
        management 110
        why the disease is an emergency? 109
    renal failure 219
    skin failure 8, 164, 174
    tubular necrosis 217
Acyclovir 213
Adrenaline
    contraindications 188
    doses 187
        adults 187
        averse effects 188
        children 188
    interactions 188
    management 188
    precaution 188
    indications 187
Adult respiratory distress syndrome 194
Airway
    access or maintenance
        complications for 142
        equipment for 139
        indications for 139
        monitoring and care of 138
        procedure for 136
    management 125
    opening of 136
Allergic interstitial nephritis 217
Aminoglycosides 218
Anaphylaxis 35, 166
    and angioedema 194

Angioedema 31, 37, 38, 40, 41, 166
Antecubital fossa 128
Antecubital vein 132
Antibacterials 216
Anticonvulsants 236
Antidotes 210
Antifungals 216
Antiphospholipid antibody syndrome 161
Approximate distribution of total body water 115
Arterial catheterization
    indications for 135
    procedure of 135
Assess platelet function 160
Atopic dermatitis 208
Atropine
    contraindication 190
    dose 190
    indications of 190
Autoimmune
    bullous disorders 197
    urticaria 198
Automated external defibrillator 149

B

Bacterial toxin mediated illness 82
    scombroid fish poisoning 88
    staphylococcal scalded skin syndrome 82
        positive Nikolsky's sign in an infant with staphylococcal scalded skin syndrome 84
        radial fissures in perioral region in a child with staphylococcal scalded skin syndrome 84
        staphylococcal scalded skin syndrome resulting in erythroderma in a child 83
    toxic shock syndrome 85
Bacteria presence 157
Barrier function of the skin 169, 174
Basic life support 149
Bedside investigations, methods of 161
Beta-lactum antibiotics 215
Betamethasone 194
Bites or stings or venom 93
    cutaneous loxoscelism (tricolor target lesion) 96
    diffuse erythema in cutaneous loxoscelism 96
    envenomation by Jellyfish 99
    spider bite (Arachnidism) 94
    tick paralysis 98

Blastocyst
    ectoderm 232
    endoderm 232
    mesoderm 232
Blister fluid of autoimmune bullous disorders 116
Blood culture
    indications for 157
    sample collection
        principles of 157
        technique of 158
Blood
    sampling 128
    volume of 126
Body fluid compartments 115
Bone marrow transplant 213
Bullous dermatoses 173

C

Calcium gluconate
    adverse effects 193
    dose 193
    heparin 193
    indication 193
Calculation of replacement fluid 117
Carbamazepine 194
Cardiopulmonary
    resuscitation 125, 128, 149
    status 125
Cardiovascular and hemodynamic drugs
    atropine 186
    diuretic 186
    fibrinolytic agents 187
    sympathomimetics 186
Cardiovascular complications 10
Central venous
    access sites for 132
    catheterization
        complications 133
        indications 132
        procedure 132
        steps of 134
Chemoprotectant 212
Chest compressions 153
Child-Pugh class C patients 227
Chronic
    kidney disease 215
    renal failure 217
Classification of drugs according to hepatic extraction 224
Class of drugs
    analgesics 216
    antibacterials 216
    antidepressants 216
    antifungals 216
    antivirals 216
Clavicle 132
Clotting time estimation of 160
Collagen vascular disorders, acute cutaneous lupus erythematosus 55, 56
Colloids 191
Comorbidities 214
Condom drainage 148
Contraction of uterine muscles 234
Conventional orotracheal intubation 140
Corticosteroids
    adverse effects 195
    dosage range for 195
    emergency care 194
    indications 194
    precaution 195
    prevention and treatment of adverse effects due to short-term use 196
    protocol for patient monitoring during short course therapy 196
Creatinine clearance 218
Critical care set up 156
Critical care unit 128
Critically ill patients, management of 131
Crystalloid
    solutions
        dextrose solutions 191
        normal saline 191
        Ringer's lactate 191
    used
        maintain lifeline and basic hydration in a critically ill patient 191
        rapid volume replacement during hypotensive shock 191
        replenish extracellular volume in dehydration 191
Cyclophosphamide
    adverse effects 203
    contraindications 203
        management of 203
        patient monitoring 203
        relative 203
    doses 203
    indications 202
Cyclosporine A
    adjustment in special situations 199
        hepatic dysfunction 199
        hyperlipidemic patients 199
        renal disease 199
    clinical and laboratory monitoring 199
    contraindications of 199
    dosage schedule 198
    indications and contraindications 198

D

Dapsone 211
Degree of renal impairment 215
Dehydration
    mild 120
    moderate 120
    severe 120

Index

Dengue
    hemorrhagic fever 161
    shock syndrome 161
Dermatological drugs
    causing acute hepatic failure 226
        analgesics 226
        antibacterials 226
        antifungals 226
        antivirals 226
        nephrotoxicity, commonly used 217
    contraindicated during lactation 237
    therapy in patients with renal impairment 214
    whose dosage adjustment is not required in renal failure 216
Dermatological emergencies
    fluid, electrolyte and nutrition therapy 114
    nursing care in 163, 169
    procedures of 125
    techniques of 125
Dermatological intensive care unit 125, 156, 177
Dermatologists skills acquired 184
Dermatomyositis 202
Dexamethasone 194
Dextran 192
Dextrose 187
DICU
    requirements 179
    arrangements 179
    instruments and equipments 177, 180
    primary requirements 179
Diseases
    autoimmune blistering 3
    Host 6, 13, 109, 111, 112
    Kawasaki 3, 5, 38, 52, 53, 54, 55, 87, 112, 197, 206, 207, 209, 213
    prototype 177
    Reiter's 6, 7, 200
    skin 4, 8, 9, 12, 113, 169, 177, 178, 214
    systemic 55
Disseminated intravascular coagulation presence of 161
Dopamine
    administration 189
    adverse effects 189
    dose 189
    indications 189
Dorsum of
    foot 128
    hand 128
Dosage adjustment
    for drugs if GFR 220,
    for low extraction drugs 226
    of drugs in renal impairment 216
Doxepin 224
DRESS syndrome 166
Drug dosing
    in acute renal failure 219
    in dialysis 219
Drug hypersensitivity syndrome 29, 149
Drug-induced cutaneous necrosis 104
    heparin-induced skin necrosis 106
    tissue necrosis due to vasopressors 107
    warfarin or coumarin necrosis 104
Drug-induced urticaria 31
Drug prescription in lactating women 236
Drug reactions 166
Drugs in pregnancy and lactation 229
Drugs precipitating pustular psoriasis 20
    clinical presentation 29
    differential diagnosis 30
    population at risk 29
    rapid laboratory diagnostic methods 30
    why the disease is an emergency? 29
Drugs
    used for definitive treatment of a dermatological condition 187
    used in dermatological emergencies 186

E

Ectoderm 232
Electrocardiography 126, 127
Embryo and fetus 229
Emergency drugs
    acid base balance and correction of electrolytes 183
    cardiovascular and hemodynamic drugs 183
    respiratory drugs 183
Endotracheal
    intubation 143
    tube in fixed position 142
    tube insertion of 142
Enteral feeding 122
Epidermolysis bullosa, types of 172
Ergot alkaloids 236
Erythema nodosum 166
Erythroderma 15, 166, 174, 200, 202
    collodion baby 16
    infantile erythroderma due to Norwegian scabies 18
    non-bullous ichthyosiform erythroderma 16
    psoriatic erythroderma 18, 19
Erythrodermic psoriasis 209
Exanthems 166
Extensive immunobullous diseases 130
External jugular veins 128
Extracellular fluid 115, 117, 216, 230
Extracutaneous lesions 209
Extravasation of fluid 130
Eye care interventions 168

F

Femoral vein 131, 132
Fetotoxicity 233
Fixed drug eruptions 166
Fluid
- and electrolyte therapy 116, 120
- balance 169
- overload 196
- resuscitation in patients with TEN 117

Frusemide
- administration 190
- adverse effects 190
- dose 189
- drug interactions 190
- indications 189

G

Gastric intolerance 201
Gastrointestinal
- function, changes in 230
- hemorrhage 196
- motility 231

Gelatine 191
Glomerular filtration rate 215, 218, 230, 231
Glomerular injury 217
Glucorunidation 216
Glucose polymer 191

H

Hemodialysis 128
Hemodialysis and hemoperfusion 210
Hemostasis of the body 163
Heparin-induced thrombocytopenia 193
Hepatic drugs clearance
- hepatic blood flow 224
- metabolism and biliary excretion 224
- protein binding of drugs 224

Herpes simplex virus 213
High binding to albumin 227
High extraction drugs 224
Human serum albumin 192
Hydrocortisone 187, 104
Hydrolyzed collagen 191
Hyperglycemia 196
Hypoalbuminemia 215
Hypotensive shock 194

I

Ichthyosis 121
Immunoablative high dose cyclophosphamide 212
Immunoablative IV, cyclophosphamide use of 212
Immunosuppressives 187
Induction of hepatic enzymes 231
Infection

Infections 67
- advanced stage of necrotizing fasciitis 68
- causes of 156
- cellulitis complicated with early changes of necrotizing fasciitis 68
- characteristic rose-red maculopapular rash of rickettsial spotted fever 77
- control of 163
- disseminated gonococcal infection 74
- meningococcemia 67, 70, 79, 81, 87
- necrotizing fasciitis 67
- petechial rash of rickettsial spotted fever over face and pinna 78
- purpura fulminans in a case of meningococcal meningitis 73
- rickettsial spotted fever 76
- spontaneous gum bleeding in a child with dengue hemorrhagic fever 81

Infliximab 209
Insensible water loss 115
Intensive care unit (ICU)
- cardiac 163, 177
- concept of 177
- neonatal 177
- neuro-medical 177
- pediatric 177

Intermediate extraction drugs 224
Internal jugular vein 131, 132
Interventions general nursing 170
- nursing 174
- specific nursing 170

Intracellular edema 121
Intratubular obstruction 217
Intravenous fluids, characteristics of 192
Intravenous immunoglobulin
- adverse effects of 197
- contraindications 197
- dosage schedule 197
- indications in dermatological emergency 197
- monitoring guidelines for therapy 198

Intravenous medications, administration of 128
Intrinsic clotting system, integrity of 160
Ion trapping 233
Isodense formulas 122
Itraconazole 194

J

Jaundice 30, 77, 95

K

Kassabach-Merritt phenomenon 204
Kassabach-Merritt syndrome 161
Kawasaki disease 207, 209
Ketoconazole 194

Index

L

Laryngoscope insertion 141
Leucovorin 210
Lichenoid eruptions 166
Life saving procedures, sequence of 153
Lipophilic drugs 215
Liver disease 227
Liver function test 201
Low extraction drugs 224

M

Maintenance fluid 118
Major drug interactions 194
Malignant disease 126
Management of acute skin failure 10
Management of dermatological
    emergencies
    atropine 183
    calcium gluconate 183
    colloids and crystalloids 183
    frusemide 183
    sodium bicarbonate 183
Mantoux test 200
Meningococcemia 161
Mesna 212
Metabolic and nutritional functions 169
Metabolic disorders 100
    acrodermatitis enteropathica 101, 103
    neonatal biotin deficiency 100
Metabolism of cyclosporine 199
Methemoglobinemia 211
Methotrexate 209
    adverse effects 201
    contraindications 201
    dose 201
    drug interactions 202
    indications 200
    patient monitoring 201
    toxicity 202, 210
    treatment 202
Methylation 216
Methylprednisolone 194
Mouth to mouth breath 152
Multidisciplinary care 179
Multi-parameter monitor 127

N

Nasogastric
    access
        equipment for 144
        indications for 143
        precaution for 146
    intubation, complications of 146
    tube insertion procedures of 144
Nasotracheal intubation 143
Necrolysis 169
Neonatal and pediatric urine collectors 150
Neonatal intensive care unit 172
Nephrotoxic drugs 217
Noninvasive blood pressure 127
Nosocomial infections 156

O

Ocular herpes simplex 195
Ongoing evaporative water loss 118
    care interventions 168
    hygiene procedures 168
    sip feeding 121
Oxygen
    saturation 127
    therapy 194

P

Pain management 171
Parasympatholytic agent 190
Parenteral nutrition 128
Parenteral solution for maintenance 119
Parkland formula 117, 118
Pemphigus vulgaris 173
Perineal dermatitis 167
Peripheral venous access
    complications 130
    procedure 130
    sites of 129
Peripheral venous lines 128
Pharmacological paralysis 167
Phenytoin 194
Pityriasis rubra pilaris 200
Placental barrier 229
Plasma volume expansion 230
Prednisolone 194
Pregnancy
    category of drug prescription
        (US FDA) 235
    drug dosing 232
    physiological changes 230
    third trimester of 231
Prerenal injury 217
Prescribing drugs in lactating women 236
Pressure ulcers
    development of 165
    prevention of 165
Principal pathomechanism of ASF 8
Proposed IADVL 123
Prostatic hypertrophy 188
Protein and calorie requirement
    recommended for patients with
        TEN 122
Protein loss in acute skin failure 115
Prototype diseases 177
Proximal convoluted tubules 215
Psoriasis 19, 207
Pulse oximeter 126, 127
Pulse rate 125
Purpura fulminans 161
Pus sample collection 158

Q

Quick fix agents
    cyclosporine 206
    infliximab 206
Quinidine 188

R

Radial artery cannulation 135
Reactions in leprosy 89
    impending nerve palsy 89
    severe neuritis with nerve abscess 89
    severe type 2 reaction in leprosy 91
Refractory pemphigus 212
Rehydration 121
Reiter's disease 200
Renal drug clearance 215
    active tubular secretion 215
    glomerular filtration 215
    tubular reabsorption 215
Renal function test 201
Rescue therapy in
    cyclophosphamide induced bladder toxicity 212
    dermatology 206
    methotrexate toxicity 209
    corticosteroid 209
Respiratory
    alkalosis 230
    drugs
        aminophylline 187
        nebulization with bronchodilators 187
    rate 125
Rickettsial spotted fever 161
Rifampicin 194
Rule of nine 117, 118
Ryle's tube 121

S

Sample collection, techniques of 161
Saphenous vein 128
Scalp veins 128
Scope of dermatology 1
Selection of
    loading dose 218
    maintenance dose 218
Sepsis and thrombocytopenia 212
Serum creatinine 227
Serum sickness 33
Set up DICU 180, 181
Severe cutaneous adverse drug reactions 22
    hemorrhagic crusts on lips in a patient with Stevens-Johnson syndrome 25
    mucosal involvement in toxic epidermal necrolysis 26
    positive Nikolsky's sign in a patient with TEN 26
    Stevens Johnson syndrome 23, 24
    toxic epidermal necrolysis with widespread epidermal detachment 25
Severity of dehydration in infants and children, clinical signs of 120
Skin
    biopsy 7
    care 164
    care of the children, principles of 172
    functions 169
    protection 172
Sodium bicarbonate
    dose 192
    drug interaction 193
    indications 192
Specimen collection from skin 158
Staphylococcal scalded skin syndrome 156, 159
Stem cell transplant patients 213
Sternocleidomastoid muscle 132
Subclavian vein 131, 132
Sudden cardiac arrest 149
Syndromes
    adult respiratory distress 15
    antiphospholipid antibody 5, 38, 47, 113, 161
    Budd-Chiari 48
    catastrophic antiphospholipid antibody 3
    dengue shock 3, 5, 80, 161, 178
    drug hypersensitivity 5, 23, 29, 30, 111, 149, 194
    Kassabach Mmerritt 161, 194
    sezary 7
    staphylococcal scalded skin 5, 27, 62, 66, 82, 83
    Stevens-Johnson syndrome 114, 156, 166, 169
    toxic shock 5, 82, 85, 161
    Waterhouse-Friderichsen 70
Systemic antibiotic therapy 173

T

Temperature control 163
Temperature regulation 169
TEN fluid and electrolyte loss 117
Teratogenicity 229
Tetrahydrofolic acid 209
Thermoregulation 9
Thrombocytopenia, presence of 161
Thymidine 210
Thymidine rescues 211
Toxic
    epidermal necrolysis 117, 130, 156, 166
    shock syndrome 161

Index

Transepidermal water loss 114, 115
Transmission of various infections 126
Transurethral catheterization
    equipment for 146
    indications for 146
    procedure for 147
Triple airway maneuver 136
Tube feeding 121
Tubular reabsorption 215

U

Underlying disease 117
Urinalysis 201
Urinary
    alkalinization 210
    catheterization 128, 147
    retention 190
    tract infection 167, 202
Urine microscopy 162

V

Valacyclovir 213
Vascular access, indications of 128
Vascular disorders 38, 55
    acute urticaria and angioedema 38
    antiphospholipid antibody syndrome 47
    calciphylaxis 38, 50, 105
    Hughes syndrome 47
    Kawasaki disease 51
        fissured lips in a child 53
        perianal desquamation in a child 53
        periungual desquamation in a child 54
        mucocutaneous lymph node syndrome 51
    purpura fulminans
        in a pregnant woman suffering from varicella 46
        with geographic areas of cutaneous necrosis 45
Venesection
    equipments for 130
    procedure 131
Vesiculobullous disorders 60, 198
    bullous pemphigoid 65, 66
    genetic blistering 60
    immunobullous 62
    pemphigus foliaceus 63
    pemphigus vulgaris 64
    tense hemorrhagic bullae of bullous pemphigoid 65
Vincristine, recommended dose 204
Volume resuscitation 128

W

Water deficit 121
Waterhouse-Friderichsen syndrome 70

X

X-ray chest 7, 27, 56, 87

Y

Yellowish greasy scale 14

Z

Zidovudine 221, 223, 224